# Welcome to the *EVERYTHING*® series!

These handy, accessible books give you all you need to tackle a difficult project, gain a new hobby, comprehend a fascinating topic, prepare for an exam, or even brush up on something you learned back in school but have since forgotten.

You can read an *EVERYTHING*® book from cover to cover or just pick out the information you want from our four useful boxes: e-facts, e-ssentials, e-alerts, and e-questions. We literally give you everything you need to know on the subject, but throw in a lot of fun stuff along the way, too.

We now have well over 100 *EVERYTHING*® books in print, spanning such wide-ranging topics as weddings, pregnancy, wine, learning guitar, one-pot cooking, managing people, and so much more. When you're done reading them all, you can finally say you know *EVERYTHING*®!

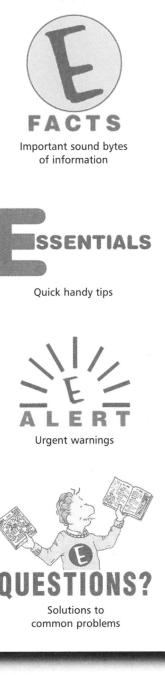

**FACTS**
Important sound bytes of information

**ESSENTIALS**
Quick handy tips

**ALERT**
Urgent warnings

**QUESTIONS?**
Solutions to common problems

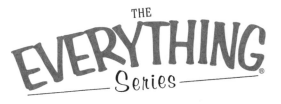

Dear Reader,

How many times in your life have you said that you wanted to lose weight? Isn't dieting a part of the American culture? Or maybe it just seems to be.

We all want to be thin and trim. We strive to look like the latest supermodel and fit into the hottest clothes. And we will do almost anything to get there, even sacrifice our health at times.

Diets in books and magazines, weight loss medications, exercise equipment, weight-reducing gadgets, products and creams . . . there are so many avenues to help us lose, so what's wrong? Why can't we lose this extra weight?

As a registered dietitian, I hear people every day telling me that they want to lose weight, that they need to lose weight and will do anything and everything to lose that weight. The problem is that people will do anything and everything except to choose the healthiest way of achieving their goal.

I wrote *The Everything® Dieting Book* to help people realize once and for all how they can lose weight successfully. It all boils down to a healthy approach to eating a variety of foods, balancing food choices, and doing so in moderation. All foods are allowed. Three meals and various snacks are allowed. Isn't this what we want? No deprivation, no restricted foods, no temporary solutions.

We all need to realize that being healthy and maintaining a healthy weight for our body size is our primary goal. Guidance found throughout the book helps you do just that. Give me a chance to help you. This may be the last "diet" you every try.

Good luck and healthy eating for life.

Sandra K Nissenberg

# THE
EVERYTHING DIETING BOOK

## Quick and easy ways to lose weight and feel great

Sandra K. Nissenberg, M.S., R.D.

Adams Media Corporation
Avon, Massachusetts

EDITORIAL
Publishing Director: Gary M. Krebs
Managing Editor: Kate McBride
Copy Chief: Laura MacLaughlin
Acquisitions Editor: Bethany Brown,
Allison Carpenter Yoder
Development Editors: Michael Paydos,
Elizabeth Kuball
Production Editor: Khrysti Nazzaro

PRODUCTION
Production Director: Susan Beale
Production Manager: Michelle Roy Kelly
Series Designer: Daria Perreault
Cover Design: Paul Beatrice and Frank Rivera
Layout and Graphics: Colleen Cunningham,
Rachael Eiben, Michelle Roy Kelly,
Daria Perreault, Erin Ring

Published by Adams Media Corporation
57 Littlefield Street, Avon, MA 02322 U.S.A.
*www.adamsmedia.com*

ISBN: 1-58062-663-7
Printed in the United States of America.

J  I  H  G  F  E  D  C  B  A

**Library of Congress Cataloging-in-Publication Data**
Nissenberg, Sandra K.
The everything dieting book/Sandra K. Nissenberg.
p.      cm.      --    (An everything series book)
ISBN 1-58062-663-7
1. Reducing diets. 2. Weight loss. I. Title. II. Everything series
RM222.2 .N575  2002
613.2'5–dc21            2002010124

This book is intended as a reference volume only, not as a medical manual. The information given here is designed to help you make informed decisions about your health. It is not intended as a substitute for any treatment that may have been prescribed by your doctor. If you suspect that you have a medical problem, we urge you to seek competent medical help.

This publication is designed to provide accurate and authoritative information with regard to the subject matter covered. It is sold with the understanding that the publisher is not engaged in rendering legal, accounting, or other professional advice. If legal advice or other expert assistance is required, the services of a competent professional person should be sought.
—From a *Declaration of Principles* jointly adopted by a Committee of the American Bar Association and a Committee of Publishers and Associations

Illustrations by Barry Littmann and Eulala Conner.
Digital illustrations courtesy of Argosy Publishing.

*This book is available at quantity discounts for bulk purchases.*
*For information, call 1-800-872-5627.*

**Visit the entire Everything® series at everything.com**

# Contents

# Introduction

THE WEIGHT-LOSS INDUSTRY IS BIG BUSINESS. Just look around and you'll see why. Articles about losing weight are the preferred topic among women's magazines. Losing weight tops New Year's resolution lists each year. Hundreds of weight-loss books are published each year and many are number one bestsellers. Fitness clubs are a primary attraction, especially at the beginning of the year. Weight-loss gadgets and equipment are hot commodities. And weight-loss drugs and products are a common request from doctors and pharmacists.

People all over the country want to lose weight. But with all the interest and attraction to weight-loss information, medications, equipment, gadgets, and products, have we seen any significant results in the weight of the American population? Are any of these things working? Year after year, we see more products and services relating to dieting and weight loss, but are we any better than we were a year ago, or even ten years ago? Actually, if you can believe it, we are worse off.

Why are we so obsessed with weight? We talk about it, read about it, see what's around us, and dwell on what we could and should be doing. We can talk, read, and wish all we want about how thin we want to be, but unless we take appropriate action, we will end up no better off than we were before.

You have to understand that dieting and exercise are not fun tasks for the majority of people. No matter how much you've tried, nothing can change you unless you are willing to make the proper changes yourself. There is no magic answer, no magic solution, pill, product, or book that will do the trick. So why wait and hang on to these fantasies any longer?

The real facts are known. When it comes to weight loss, we know what works and what does not work. Many people just don't want to face the truth. Losing weight takes time. It takes planning, and it takes change. But since we do know what works, why not make the decision now, once and for all, to do something about your weight? Time will continue to pass. Don't waste any more of it. It is time to take action now.

This book offers everything you want, and need, to know about dieting and losing that excess weight once and for all. At the same time, it shows you how to keep a healthy prospective while you accomplish your goal. It is written to be an authentic source of helpful and long-lasting information. Direction on eating for life is the goal. No more restrictive diets. No more short-term, temporary solutions. The time is now to focus on achieving and maintaining a healthy lifestyle by creating a lifelong approach to changing habits, changing attitudes, and changing yourself for good. Good luck and healthy eating!

## CHAPTER 1
# *Facing the Weight Challenge*

Millions of people each year want to lose weight. They want to lose it fast, painlessly, and to keep it off forever. The problem is that so many people want that quick and magic diet, pill, or potion. So few are really willing to sit back, educate themselves properly, and create a program of healthy, long-term weight loss. Why?

# Overweight Versus Obesity

In years past, being overweight and even obese was a sign of prosperity and wealth. The more prosperity and wealth we had, the better we ate and the more corpulent we looked. Today, we look at body weight in just the opposite way. The smarter we are, the richer we are, the more visible we are, the thinner we want to be. We feel that our weight reflects on us as a person. Excess weight makes us look as though we don't take care of ourselves. When did this attitude change?

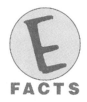

**FACTS**

At any one time in the United States, more than 50 percent of the women and more than 25 percent of the men consider themselves to be on a diet.

We often use the terms *overweight* and *obesity* interchangeably in speaking, but in fact they are quite different in meaning. An overweight person is defined as one who carries extra weight in the form of muscles, bones, water, and fat. An overweight person could be a competitive athlete who may have increased muscle mass or a person with short stature who may have a large bone structure. On the other hand, an obese person has an excess of body fat only. His or her weight is found in extra fat stores throughout various parts of the body.

Currently it is estimated that almost 40 million Americans are obese—about one-third of all adults and one in five children. More than 50 percent of our entire population is considered overweight. As a result of this high incidence, obesity is reported to contribute to at least 300,000 excess deaths in this country and hundreds of million dollars in health care costs each year.

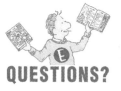

**QUESTIONS?**

**What is the difference between overweight and obesity?**
Overweight is the result of an excess of body weight that accumulates from body tissues like muscle, bone, fat, or water while an obesity state comes from the excess of body fat alone.

# So Why Lose Weight?

Yes, we are obsessed with losing weight. But are there good reasons to take off those extra pounds. People who are obese and overweight can gain significant benefits from losing weight—even small amounts, as little as 10 to 20 pounds.

For individuals who are overweight or obese, losing weight should be an important goal in health. It's not just considered a cosmetic concern. But just as important is maintaining the weight loss. Keeping your weight to ideal conditions for your size helps in disease prevention and in seeking a state of overall well-being.

## The Risks of Being Obese

Here is what we know about the risks of being obese:

- Being obese puts people at risk for some types of cancer, for diabetes, heart disease, stroke, arthritis, gall bladder disease, and hypertension (high blood pressure)—some of which are leading causes of death in America today.
- Being obese adds stress to the body; extra weight makes your body work harder to function—it becomes harder to breathe, move, and keep the heart beating normally.
- Being obese causes depression; it is not uncommon to find many obese persons who are depressed about life in general.
- Being obese is unattractive; it's harder to find clothes, feel good in clothes, and have others admire you as well.
- Being obese reduces your self-esteem; it causes people of all ages to have a low opinion about themselves.
- Being obese may cause discrimination; obese individuals can face discrimination at work, school, and socially, too.

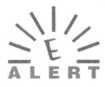

The Surgeon General reports that the risk of premature death rises with increased weight gain, even in as much as 10–20 pounds for an individual of average height.

## Obesity As a Disease

Until recently, obesity in a person was thought of as a sign of the person's lack of willpower. It was a stigma assigned to people who were thought to have no control over what and how much they ate. People who carried excess weight were ridiculed for putting it on and keeping it on. Although many people still feel this way, medical experts now categorize obesity as a disease, just like heart disease, diabetes, high blood pressure, and cancer. It's a disease that many people have no control over.

Recent efforts by medical experts and the National Institutes of Health have labeled obesity as a disease—a disease that has problems generated from genetics, the environment, and psychological factors. And along with obesity being a disease in itself, it is known to lead to other chronic diseases, including heart disease, stroke, diabetes, gall bladder disease, arthritis, high blood pressure, and some forms of cancer. All of these chronic conditions can lead to illness and even premature death.

But I'm not saying that everyone needs to be slim, trim, and the size of a model. In fact, for many individuals who *do not* need to lose weight, losing weight offers no health benefit and can often be more harmful than helpful. But for those who do need to lose the weight, losing even 10, 20, or 30 pounds can bring on tremendous health benefits—decreasing blood pressure, reducing blood glucose levels, lowering cholesterol, increasing self esteem, and even bringing on a sense of accomplishment.

# How Your Shape Affects Health Risk

Every person is shaped differently. Two people can be the same height and the same weight and yet be built in totally different ways. Your size, your shape, and how you carry your excess pounds can increase or decrease your health risks due to obesity.

## Apple Versus Pear

Where a person carries his excess weight is a determinant of overall health risk. Men or women who store fat around their stomach or middle portion of the body are at greater risk of complications than those who carry weight on their hips, thighs, or buttocks. This is largely because the fat accumulation around the vital bodily organs is more critical than that which accumulates around the legs and thighs. Often compared to the shape of an apple or a pear, body shapes are important in assessing future risk of obesity-related health concerns.

## Waist-to-Hip Ratio

You can determine where your fat accumulates and if you are shaped more like an apple or a pear by calculating your waist-to-hip ratio. Measure your waist at the narrowest spot. Then measure your hips at the widest spot. Divide the inches from the waist measurement by the inches of the hip measurement. For example, a person with a 38-inch waist and 40-inch hips would calculate her ratio like so: 38 divided by 40 = 0.95. A person with a 30-inch waist and 40-inch hips would calculate as 30 divided by 40 = 0.75. Women with ratios lower than 0.80 and men with ratios lower than 1.0 are considered "pear-shaped." Women who have a ratio greater than 0.80 and men who have a ratio of greater than 1.0 are considered "apple-shaped." They are therefore at greater health risk due to their body shape and fat distribution.

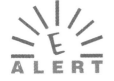

The number of overweight children and teens has risen more than 200 percent in the last decade.

# Other Factors Affecting Risk of Obesity

Besides health-related issues, there are many other factors that can contribute to obesity in our society. Not only are adults feeling greater effects of being overweight, our younger generation of children and teens have never been heavier.

Gadgets like the remote control, garage door openers, computers, and video games are just some of the contributing factors. People just don't have to move anymore to do what they need to do and get what they need to get. Kids are not as active as they used to be. Transportation is available everywhere. School physical education programs are limited in many schools around the country. And the abundance of fast foods, convenience foods, and frequent snacks tends to cause additional weight gain at younger and younger ages.

Poor eating habits of parents also lead to poor eating habits of children. Habits are shared and passed on from generation to generation. As a result, children are becoming more overweight than ever before. Their risk rises with obese parents, and even more so with obese siblings.

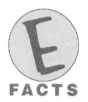

**FACTS**

It is estimated that children of two obese parents have an 80 percent likelihood of becoming obese, as compared to only about 15 percent if both parents are of average weight.

## What Causes Obesity?

The majority of people become obese from consuming more food than their body needs or using up less energy than their body takes in. This can result from eating too much, exercising too little, or a combination of both.

### Heredity and Genetic Factors

For a small number of individuals, heredity and genetic factors could come into play. Genetic factors can result in endocrine problems from an underactive thyroid, meaning a person's metabolism is slower than it should be. But even though many people may want to *believe* this is their problem, this is most often the exception rather than the rule. Although it's not uncommon for obesity to run in families, it's most likely that a combination of genetics with lifestyle and eating habits are to blame.

### Environmental Factors

A person's environment also can contribute to obesity. If an individual lives in a home where large meals and sedentary living are the norm, it's likely that their habits will follow suit. And, of course, your overall size may be a factor in extra weight gain. Some people have a tendency toward a short stature due to their genetics. These individuals have a smaller body mass to feed and as a result this may lead to weight problems if they often eat like their taller, larger counterparts.

## Balancing the Equation

What we know about gaining weight is simple: What goes in must be balanced with what goes out. **FIGURE 1-2** shows a simple illustration.

**FIGURE 1-2:**
Weight
Maintenance

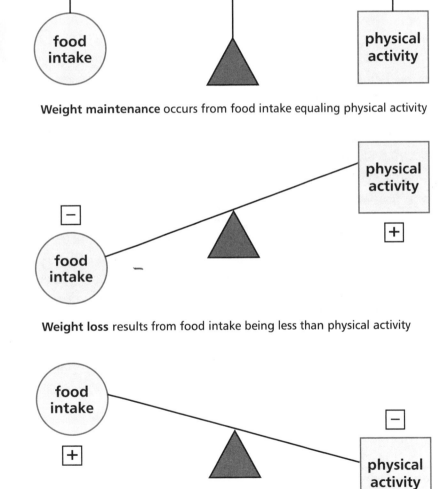

Weight maintenance occurs from food intake equaling physical activity

Weight loss results from food intake being less than physical activity

Weight gain results from food intake being greater than physical activity

# Where Do Eating Habits Come From?

Eating habits result from a learned behavior that is practiced over and over again. These are often difficult to break because they have been repeated over and over again for years. Some examples of eating habits include drinking coffee every morning, having dessert after a meal, or munching on popcorn during a movie.

People form habits from their infant years as they are taught by their parents and caregivers—their role models. The types of foods, where these foods are eaten, snack choices, and exercise patterns are all habits formed early in life. Good habits are as easy to create as bad ones are, but if parents reinforce unhealthy habits, usually meaning if they practice these habits themselves, it is likely that these habits will be passed on to younger generations as well. Parents also serve as their children's role models through the growing years and help their children get on the path toward their own independent lifestyles. If good patterns are not taught early, they are difficult to pick up later.

Eating habits can change throughout life—for the better and also for the worse. Busy schedules, family food preferences, peer pressure, and fast-paced lifestyles often create habits of skipping meals, consuming frequent convenience and fast foods, finishing a child's plate, eating on the run, and eating whether hungry or not. But on the contrary, having children in your home may inspire you to prepare a family breakfast or try new fruit and vegetable selections at the grocery store or even plan a festive (and healthy) dinner party.

**E**SSENTIALS

Obesity runs in families not only because family members share the same genes, but because they also share the same lifestyle habits.

Whatever your initial goal may be in aiming to find a more desirable weight, I'm going to help you learn what you can do, how you can change, and what and how you should be eating.

# Evaluating Your Lifestyle

First, begin by examining yourself and evaluating your lifestyle and food-style trends. Put a check mark in the appropriate column.

## HOW'S MY LIFESTYLE

| | ALWAYS | OCCASIONALLY | NEVER |
|---|---|---|---|
| I eat regular meals and snacks daily (at least three meals and one to two snacks/day). | ❑ | ❑ | ❑ |
| I eat breakfast every day. | ❑ | ❑ | ❑ |
| I eat a variety of foods from each food group (breads/cereals, fruits, vegetables, dairy, meat/protein) daily. | ❑ | ❑ | ❑ |
| I eat at least six grains or grain products daily, choosing primarily whole grains. | ❑ | ❑ | ❑ |
| I eat at least three different vegetables each day. | ❑ | ❑ | ❑ |
| I consume at least three different varieties of fruit or juice each day. | ❑ | ❑ | ❑ |
| I consume at least two servings of low-fat dairy products daily. | ❑ | ❑ | ❑ |
| I eat lean beef, chicken, fish, eggs, or legumes twice daily. | ❑ | ❑ | ❑ |
| I limit my intake of high-fat and high-sugar foods. | ❑ | ❑ | ❑ |
| I choose many high-fiber foods each day. | ❑ | ❑ | ❑ |
| I choose healthy, nutritious snack foods. | ❑ | ❑ | ❑ |
| I drink at least six cups of water (or clear fluids) daily. | ❑ | ❑ | ❑ |
| I get at least twenty minutes of physical activity three to four times each week. | ❑ | ❑ | ❑ |
| I get at least six to seven hours of sleep each night. | ❑ | ❑ | ❑ |
| I limit alcoholic beverages to no more than one each day. | ❑ | ❑ | ❑ |
| I try to eat out no more than three times each week. | ❑ | ❑ | ❑ |

Now, look at your check marks. If you really are on top of your lifestyle, you will have checked off all answers in the "always" column. This is your aim. Here, this would mean you have a very healthy lifestyle and very good habits. If you have several marked off in the "always" column and several in the "occasionally" column, you're on your way to a better lifestyle. If, by chance, you marked any answers in the "never" column, you need to make some changes. I'm here to help you do just that.

# Making Permanent Changes

We all do it. It's human nature to put off things we do not like to do—like studying for an exam, finishing a home-improvement project, or starting to watch our weight. We can always find an excuse. It is now time to make this time different.

You picked up this book to help yourself accomplish a goal. Whether you want to educate yourself about dieting, change your eating style, or both, I am here to help. Your first plan of action is to set some initial goals.

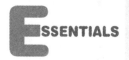
**ESSENTIALS**

Heredity factors may determine the upper and lower limits of your body weight, but a combination of lifestyle factors keeps you up and down within those limits.

## Setting Goals

Let's say your primary goal is to lose 20 pounds. This can be your long-term goal. Now how are you going to manage this weight loss? Change food habits, begin a walking program, purchase new varieties of fruits and vegetables, prepare more meals at home—each of these are short-term goals that can help accomplish your long-term plans.

## Long-Term and Short-Term Goals

Success of any type is built on establishing long-term and short-term goals—goals that are realistic and challenging. Long-term goals help you imagine where you want to be a year from now. Short-term goals set your plans for the upcoming week or month. These are more realistic goals that are easily attainable. If you make these short-term goals weekly, one each week, you can bring on over fifty changes in one year. Or if you prefer, try one each month and incorporate twelve in a year. And I'm talking about small changes. These small-term changes help you meet and accomplish these long-term goals.

To help you along, here are several more examples. Long-term goals should not be impossible to meet, but should add a challenge, like these:

- I want to get in good enough shape to run a marathon.
- I want to go on a two-day, 100-mile bike race.
- I want to wear a size ten by next summer.

Short-terms goals should be those that can be met without a great deal of effort. These short-term accomplishments help reinforce that changes can be made while motivating you to continue striving for success, like these:

- I will walk for fifteen minutes each day.
- I will stop eating and snacking after 8:00 P.M.
- I will eat breakfast at least three mornings each week.
- I will put out a fruit basket each day with different varieties of fruit to try.
- I will cut down the amount of soft drinks I drink to one each day.

**FACTS**

Just losing an initial 10 to 20 pounds can bring on physical and psychological benefits to make you feel better, be healthier, and be more motivated to continue.

## Your Own Personal Goals

Now it is time for you to set some initial goals for yourself. Ask yourself the following questions:

- What do I want to accomplish in the next year?
- What do I want to accomplish in the next month to help meet this goal?
- What do I want to accomplish in the next week to help meet this goal?

Now it is time to get started. You have identified the need to lose some weight and decided it's time to start once and for all. You've determined you are ready to start, to set some initial goals for yourself, and that you are ready for success, not failure.

As we continue, I want you to realize that I am here to help you make long-term lifestyle changes, ones that can last a lifetime. Keep in mind that attempts to lose weight are not temporary. "Dieting" is not a temporary state. Losing and maintaining a healthy weight is something you want to do for you, not for your mother, not for your spouse, and not for your best friend. It is a lifelong effort that takes education, determination, and a will to be as healthy as you can be.

## CHAPTER 2

# *What Should I Weigh?*

**A**ll throughout life people focus on their body weight. When they were little, they wanted to weigh more. When they get older, they want to weigh less. Is there any happy medium to this madness? Why do people get so absorbed in these numbers?

# The Benefits and Limitations of the Bathroom Scale

The bathroom scale is the most common tool people use to help determine their body weight. This scale is often taken too seriously and, of course, it is one of the most hated tools used on a regular basis. Over and over again people continue to "torture" themselves by weighing in, while constantly complaining about the dreaded results.

**ESSENTIALS**  The bathroom scale is a useful tool for marking and charting body weight, but it does not take into consideration bone structure, muscle mass, genetics, or other factors that contribute to weight.

How do you feel about your scale? Are you too focused on your body weight? Ask yourself the following questions:

- Do you weigh first thing every morning and then again sometimes at night, too?
- Do you weigh yourself more than three times each week, either at home or away?
- Do you judge yourself by the numbers you see on the scale?
- Does your weight for the day determine your day's demeanor?
- Do you often dwell on the number you see on the scale?
- Do you swear or curse at the scale because the numbers disappoint you?
- Do you often insist on dropping a few pounds until you will buy yourself a new outfit?
- Do you constantly discuss your desire to lose weight with others?

If you answered yes to two or more of these questions, you are not alone, but you need to think more clearly about your relationship with your scale and particularly with your body weight. Too many of us define ourselves by a particular number and think less of ourselves if we don't meet our expectations. Are you spending too much energy worrying about your weight?

Whether or not you choose to use the bathroom scale on a regular basis, it still remains your most accessible tool for determining body weight. If and when you do use your scale, do so with the following tips in mind for the most accurate results:

- **Use the same scale.** Different scales may present different results. Also be sure the scale sits on a "flat" floor, not carpeting.
- **Weigh yourself no more than one time each week.** Select the same day, same time. Body weight can fluctuate. The best way to evaluate your body weight is to weigh yourself in the morning, preferably before you have eaten, and without clothing.
- **Stand straight in the middle of the scale.** Your scale can record different numbers based on where and how you stand on it. You will get the best and most accurate readings by standing straight up and with your feet planted in the center.
- **Understand body changes.** Menstrual cycles, sodium intake, and medications can all influence water retention and, therefore, water and body weight. Keep this in mind if you notice rapid, unwelcome increases.

# Understanding Body Weight

Too many Americans are preoccupied with their body weight. More than half of all women and more than one-third of men are dissatisfied with their shape, size, or body weight. And these obsessions are even higher among our younger population. In many cases, people see themselves as much worse off than others see them. What can we do about this?

## Is Body Weight Constant Throughout Life?

There are so many people who focus on a set body weight based on the chart found on the wall of the doctor's office or illustrated in a book. Some believe that this number is set in stone and that it should not vary throughout adult life. They think that their body weight in their twenties should remain constant through their thirties, forties, and beyond.

Focusing on a set number can be the first step in developing an obsession with body weight that can continue throughout life. Too many times, people dwell on what they weighed when they got married or before they had a child. (Isn't it funny how we can clearly remember these numbers?) This obsession can take over your life and can lead to problems with health, depression, and your overall well-being.

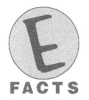

**FACTS**

American society places way too much emphasis on body weight and size. Messages are hard for most people to take, whether they are within healthy weight ranges or not. You need to understand who you are as a person, on the inside, and not focus solely on your outside appearance. In the meantime, aim for a healthier attitude. Instead of seeking to be thin, focus on being healthy.

## Who Decides What's Ideal?

Old measurements for determining an "ideal" weight for a person were based on the height/weight charts compiled by an insurance company. Tables were established based on height and weight ratios of insured persons with the greatest lifespan. Two charts were generally used, one for those nineteen to thirty-four and another for those thirty-five and older. People looked up their height and age on these charts. The charts gave a range in which their weights should fall, with the midpoint being that person's "ideal."

Over the years, health researchers and nutrition professionals determined height/weight chart measurements were not as accurate as they could be and that these numbers did not take into account optimal body composition, including fat distribution. Many people swore by the numbers on the chart, but in fact these were not always the best measurement of our population as a whole.

## Determining a Healthy Weight

A healthy weight is a range for a particular body build that takes into account total fat, muscle, bone, and water for a person's size. This weight varies from person to person and is established to be the weight somewhere between an underweight status and an overweight status, at which this person would be most healthy.

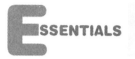

**SSENTIALS**

Healthy weight should not be confused with a weight in which a person is his or her slimmest or thinnest.

## Healthy Weight Versus Normal/Ideal Weight

Today, standards regarding weight have changed. Many health professionals prefer to use the term "healthy weight" rather than referring to one's "normal" or "ideal" weight. A "healthy" weight depends on a number of factors—age, gender, height, and frame or body size.

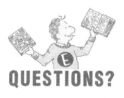

**QUESTIONS?**

**Does every person have a predetermined weight?**
Some researchers believe so. This predetermined weight, often referred to as a person's "set point," implies that each person may have a predestined weight that allows a variation of about 10 percent on each side. For most individuals, staying within this range is quite easy, but moving beyond it is difficult.

Charts created recently more accurately take into account total body composition. They do so by providing ranges of numbers that are appropriate for individuals, rather than just a single number. Because no one person stays at the same weight for his entire life, and because bodies change through the years, no one weight is standard for a person during his entire life. It is very common for women to add an extra 10 to 15 pounds, and for men to gain 20 to 30 pounds, throughout their adult years. And it is healthy to do so. During one's elder years, when illnesses or accidents may be more common, a few extra pounds can be a benefit by providing additional stores of body fat and some extra cushioning around the bones.

## Healthy Weight Ranges for Adults

One such established chart helps individuals determine a "healthy weight range" for themselves. This chart takes a range of numbers into account, not just a single one, thereby allowing higher numbers for those people with larger body builds and greater amounts of muscle and bone. This chart is also useful for all adult age groups. While it is believed that people put on weight as they age, this weight gain should remain within the allowable range for height.

| HEIGHT IN FEET/INCHES (WITHOUT SHOES) | WEIGHT IN POUNDS (WITHOUT CLOTHES) |
|---|---|
| 4'10" | 91–119 |
| 4'11" | 94–124 |
| 5'0" | 97–128 |
| 5'1" | 101–132 |
| 5'2" | 104–137 |
| 5'3" | 107–141 |
| 5'4" | 111–146 |
| 5'5" | 114–150 |
| 5' 6" | 118–155 |
| 5'7" | 121–160 |
| 5'8" | 125–164 |
| 5'9" | 129–169 |
| 5'10" | 132–174 |
| 5'11" | 136–179 |
| 6'0" | 140–184 |
| 6'1" | 144–189 |
| 6'2" | 148–195 |
| 6'3" | 152–200 |
| 6'4" | 156–205 |
| 6'5" | 160–211 |
| 6'6" | 164–216 |

This chart can also be illustrated to demonstrate ranges for determining moderate and severe overweight status as well.

**FIGURE 2-1:**
Healthy
weight ranges

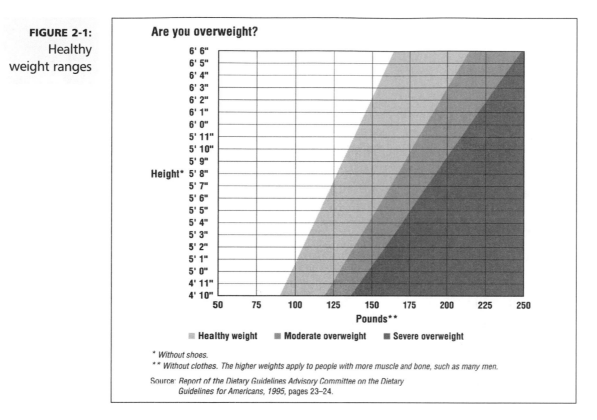

**Are you overweight?**

* Without shoes.
** Without clothes. The higher weights apply to people with more muscle and bone, such as many men.

Source: *Report of the Dietary Guidelines Advisory Committee on the Dietary Guidelines for Americans, 1995*, pages 23–24.

# Determining Body Fat

Most people have used height/weight tables at one time or another. Health professionals often question their effectiveness but understand their basic purpose. These charts help primarily in determining whether a person falls into a healthy weight or not. More accurate measures are available, and are currently used, that take into account how much body fat a person has.

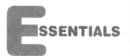

**SSENTIALS**

Height/weight charts can be limiting and should not be taken as an indication of overall health status. Body size is not the important issue—body composition is.

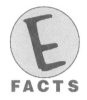

**FACTS**

Men are considered obese when more than 25 percent of their weight is body fat whereas women are considered obese when more than 30 percent of weight is body fat.

Everybody needs a certain amount of fat in his or her body for energy sources, heat insulation, shock absorption, and various other vital functions. Women, for the most part, have greater fat stores than men. Precisely determining how much body fat a person has is a difficult and somewhat costly process. Several options are available, but in order to obtain accurate results, trained professionals and expensive equipment are often necessary.

## Underwater Weighing

One of the most effective ways to accurately measure lean muscle versus fat weight is through underwater (hydrostatic) weighing. Underwater weighing takes place by submerging a person into a tank of water about four feet deep as air is forced out of the person's lungs. After staying underwater for about six to ten seconds, the person's weight is recorded. This method is based on the principles that people with greater muscle mass weigh more in water than those who do not and that fat floats in water. Therefore, more accurate measures of lean body mass can be recorded underwater. This process is repeated up to five to ten times. An average is then recorded and calculated according to a special formula to determine the percentage of total fat weight. This method of determining body fat can be costly and is not widely available to most people.

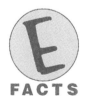

**FACTS**

The majority of women store fat in their hips, buttocks, thighs, and breasts whereas men primarily store their weight in their abdomens, lower back, and chests.

## Bioelectrical Impedance Analysis

Another fat-measurement method, called *bioelectrical impedance analysis*, is a relatively new and simple method. This process can determine overall body fat by providing a computerized calculation of lean weight, standard weight-range measurements, and percentage of body fat by delivering a harmless, low-voltage electrical current throughout the body.

This method produces an estimate of total body water and of lean muscle mass, which contains water. Water is known as an excellent conductor of electricity, while fat is known to contain very little water and is therefore resistant to the electrical flow. The more body fat a person has, the more resistance there will be to the flow of the electrical current. From this measure of resistance, a percentage of body fat is determined. Again, although this method demonstrates accuracy, it is quite expensive and is not widely available for use by most people.

## Skinfold Measurement Testing

A simpler, more common measurement of fatness in a body can be made through using skinfold calipers. These calipers are the most economical and the easiest tool to use to determine body fat composition. Trained individuals use this special tool to help determine the amount of body fat that lies just beneath the skin. This fat, called *subcutaneous fat*, ac-counts for almost half of the body's overall fat supply. The process of testing involves taking a skinfold measurement of the thickness at various points of the body, typically the upper arm, upper back, lower back, abdomen, and thigh. The amount of subcutaneous fat found in these areas helps determine the total amount of fat that can be found throughout the body. This method is widely available at many health and fitness clubs and by physicians and dietitians, and it offers an effective means of proper measurement.

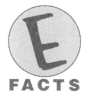

FACTS

Subcutaneous fat lies just beneath the skin and accounts for approximately half of all the fat in the body. When skinfold measurements are taken on the thigh, upper arm, abdomen and/or back, the amount of fat found in these areas helps determine the total amount of fat found throughout the body.

## Body Pinch Test

There are several other options for individuals to seek a quick and easy measurement of their own body fat. One is a simplified method of the skinfold caliper method, known as the *body pinch test*. You can easily do this yourself. Grasp the skin below the upper arm, halfway between the shoulder and elbow, and again at an inch below the waist. The skin, not the muscle, should be pinched with the thumb and forefinger. Take a measurement of the amount of skin grabbed. If the measurement is greater than an inch, an indication of an excess body fat can be made. The old slogan "pinch-an-inch" was derived from this body pinch test.

## Waist Measurement

You can also assess your health risk from your waist measurement. Here you would be measuring the amount of excess fat around your middle, or around the vital organs in the body. A waist measurement of greater than 35 inches for women and 40 inches for men indicates a risk to overall health status.

## New Methods on the Horizon

New methods of determining body fat levels are continuing to be researched and developed. Some may require expensive equipment, while others can be found in products similar to the bathroom scale. As more options become available, individuals will have greater access to these testing methods.

## Guidelines for Body Fat Determination

Each of these processes provides a person with his or her percentage of body fat. Guidelines established to determine healthy levels based on percentage of body fat are as follows:

|  | NORMAL/HEALTHY | OVERWEIGHT | OBESE |
|---|---|---|---|
| Women | 15 to 25 percent | 25.1 to 29.9 percent | greater than 30 percent |
| Men | 10 to 20 percent | 20.1 to 24.9 percent | greater than 25 percent |

Keep in mind that everyone needs some fat in their bodies to store energy, help with heat insulation, and perform other necessary functions. Women's bodies contain more fat than men's bodies do; women also have less muscle and bone than men.

# Body Mass Index

Widely used today, a common and somewhat simple tool for comparing body weight and height to body fat can be calculated by determining a person's body mass index (BMI).

## What Is the Body Mass Index?

Developed in 1993 by the National Institute of Diabetes and Digestive and Kidney Disorders, the BMI uses a mathematical formula and chart designated to correlate body weight and height to overall body fat. Federal guidelines now use the BMI guidelines to define weight groups among Americans. Although BMI figures are not an appropriate weight evaluation tool for everyone, they are more accurate than the original height/weight tables. There are several simpler ways in which you can determine your BMI.

## Calculating Your Own BMI

Body mass index can be determined in a number of ways. Some ways are simpler than others. The determination of BMI is derived from the ratio of body weight in kilograms to height in meters squared. You can determine your own BMI by dividing your weight in pounds by the square of your height in inches, like so:

1. Divide your weight in pounds by 2.2 to get your weight in kilograms.
2. Divide your height in inches by 39.37 to get your height in meters.
3. Multiply the number you got in Step 2 (your height in meters) times itself.
4. Divide the number you got in Step 1 (your weight in kilograms) by the number you got in Step 3 (height in meters × height in meters).

The result is your BMI. Here's an example, using a 150-pound female, who is 5 feet 4 inches tall. In the first step, she would divide 150 by 2.2 to get 68.18. In the second step, she would divide her height in inches (64) by 39.37, to get 1.63 meters. In the third step, she would multiply her height in meters times itself ($1.63 \times 1.63$), to get 2.66. And in the fourth step, she would divide 68.18 by 2.66, to get a BMI of 25.63.

Another more simplified formula can also be used without converting pounds into kilograms and inches into meters. Your final results will be very similar to the results found above. Try this formula now: weight in pounds multiplied by 704.5, divided by (height in inches times height in inches) = BMI. So 150 pounds $\times$ 704.5 divided by ($64 \times 64$) = BMI, or 105,675 divided by 4,096 = BMI of 25.79.

## BMI Charts

A method for determining BMI at a glance helps people estimate their BMI by drawing a line from their height in inches (on the left) across to meet their weight in pounds. Their BMI is the number at which these numbers meet. There are many other charts designed to determine your BMI at a glance. There are also many BMI calculators available on the Internet—visit *www.nhlbi.nih.gov/guidelines/obesity/bmi_tbl2.htm* for a good example.

## Evaluating Your Results

Whatever means you decide to use to determine your BMI, you will need to compare your results with the key found here. This information allows you to see how you fit into the standards established for a healthy weight:

- Underweight status equals a BMI of 19 or below
- Healthy weight equals a BMI of 19.1–24.9
- Overweight status equals a BMI of 25–29.9
- Obesity status equals a BMI of 30 or more

## Limitations of the Body Mass Index

Whatever your results may be, keep in mind that BMI figures can be limiting in several regards. These charts, although primarily useful for adults, are less indicative of weight issues in the younger population groups of children and teens. For this reason, these particular charts should not be used as an indicator of weight problems in children and young teens. Other charts have been developed for children and adolescents that should be used in combination with other assessment tools. But again, it is difficult to determine numbers and cutoffs for those whose bodies are still growing. The figures can also be misleading for individuals with larger percentages of muscle mass because measurements may indicate more of an overweight status for someone who may not fall into this category.

**FACTS**

**Using BMI standards, only 41 percent of all Americans are classified at a healthy weight—39 percent of males and 44 percent of females.**

Each and every person who uses the BMI chart and figures needs to realize, again, that these figures and numbers are only guidelines. These, as well as any height/weight chart you may find and compare to yourself, should not be your only indicator of a weight concern. Primarily these guidelines are established for healthy, adult individuals, not children, pregnant women, athletes, or frail elderly. This information is primarily useful in determining personal health risks.

## Accepting Yourself for Who You Are

Concerns regarding body weight in any individual should be made to a health professional. No one should put himself or herself down for not falling into a certain number that may be unrealistic. Appropriate direction should concentrate on following a healthier lifestyle and not on just a specific number.

An assessment of a person's weight is just that: an assessment. People need to realize that numbers help in determining this assessment. Each and every person must come to terms with his own body, what he is born with, how tall or short he is, and what size or shape he may be. We all need to understand what can be changed and what cannot. Every person is different—with a different size, a different shape, and a different metabolism. Your opinion of yourself stems from how you accept your personal self. Becoming healthier is one change that you can make. It should be your main focus, not just being as thin as you can be.

And again, keep in mind that weight is only one measurement of health. A thin person may not always be healthier than an overweight person. Many factors contribute to your overall health. As we progress through these pages, I provide more information on ways for you to build a healthy lifestyle through the foods and activities you choose.

## CHAPTER 3

# *Why We Eat What We Eat*

Why do we really eat what we do? We eat for a variety of reasons. One obvious reason is to nourish our bodies, to help us live, to help us grow, and to survive. But that isn't the only reason. With the abundance of food, especially in our country, food has become, for many people, a source of comfort, joy, and happiness that is used to relieve stress, anxiety, boredom, and loneliness.

# Factors Affecting Food Choices

The foods you eat say a lot about your character, your personality, and where you are from. They can reflect family history, culture, and religious backgrounds, your economic status, how you feel, where you go, and what you do socially.

## Ethnic Influences

Eating and choosing foods is no longer just about nutrition and feeding your body what it needs and what tastes good. Eating has become wrapped up into so many other issues. Your culture is often apparent in the foods you eat. Food practices are different from culture to culture and from generation to generation. Whether your background is European or African, Asian or Latin American, these influences contribute to the foods you eat and bring into your home.

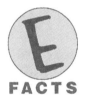

**FACTS**

Our country is a melting pot of cultures, people, and the foods we eat. You can find varieties in almost every town and city in America.

Ethnic groups influence food choices. People who share similar racial backgrounds also find themselves choosing similar foods. These influences can blend into preparation and serving methods, too. Mexican dishes often include an abundance of beans, rice, and cheese. Middle Eastern menus are known for their olives and olive oil, fruits, vegetables, and spices. Chinese foods include many stir-fry and combination meals. African-American foods, often referred to as "soul food," are commonly fried and high in fat.

## Religious Influences

Religious groups like Muslims, Seventh-Day Adventists, and Jews also can influence individual food and beverage dietary practices. Muslims are known to fast at certain times during the calendar year; many Seventh-Day Adventists follow strict vegetarian practices and avoid alcohol, coffee, and tea; and some Jews observe kosher dietary laws. People of these, and other, backgrounds may be very strict or somewhat lenient with their followings.

## Regional Influences

America is scattered with a vast amount of food choices—just as it is scattered with a vast amount of different cultures and ethnic groups. Foods can be found everywhere—grocery stores, ethnic markets, restaurants, street fairs and festivals, and from traveling in, around, and out of the country.

Along with the many cultures and ethnic groups found in our country, America has its own collection of regional food preferences. Each region of our country is known for its distinct types of foods. The wide number of ethnic heritages, national resources, and diverse types of people found throughout these regions largely contribute to these preferences.

The South originated foods like hush puppies and cheese grits. The Southwest is known for its Mexican-American foods like tacos and enchiladas. The Northeast is famous for its supply of seafood and fresh fish, and the West Coast, with its warm weather and trendy lifestyle, is where you can often find many fresh foods and Asian/Pacific-type foods.

## Social Influences

Our social existence is probably one of the biggest contributors to what we eat. The people we live with, work with, and socialize with have a great deal of influence over what we eat.

Friends, peers, and colleagues are also a big influence over food choices. Teens are notorious for eating like their friends and peers. They might choose foods like pizza, French fries, hot dogs, shakes, and soft drinks because everyone else is eating these. On the other hand they might choose to not eat at all, in order to "trim down" like their friends.

And fellow colleagues are known to make food choices for us during a coffee break or at lunch. "Let's grab a latte and doughnut," or "How about a burger and fries for lunch today?"

## Family Influence

Your family's eating and purchasing decisions provide the greatest input into your current food habits. How your parents fed you—what foods were brought into the home, how you celebrated special occasions—led to how you eat. These environmental factors have probably the largest impact on your overall food decisions today.

Modern families are different and more widely diverse than ever before. We see many more single-parent households, many homes with two working parents, and various nonfamily individuals living together. Busy schedules also reflect on eating decisions. The majority of our meals are no longer prepared from scratch and over a stove. Many nights go by without a hot meal being prepared in the home at all. The frequency of restaurant dining, fast food, and convenience dinners has eclipsed more traditional meals. The microwave has now become the favored kitchen appliance—heat it up and finish in ten minutes or less. Activities and family schedules now take priority over home-cooked meals.

# What about the Media?

How has the media led to our food intake and habits? Television, magazine, and newspaper advertisements are often a big factor in our purchasing and eating decisions. Food companies spend millions of dollars each year to influence your decisions. The more you see and read about a new product, the more you will be apt to try it. Coupons, store displays, tasting stations, and placement of a product on the grocery store shelf also encourage buyers to purchase it.

Children, too, make food decisions based on what they see on television or what they hear about from their friends. Advertisements during children's programs cater to that age group and are primarily influencing what children most request from their parents. Children today have much more influence over their food choices than in years past, and parents are often pleased to oblige.

The effect of the media on eating behaviors is enormous and can be both beneficial and harmful as well. Not only are some foods advertised as the healthy and newest variety available, but other "not-so-healthy" choices frequently pop up, too. The media also overvalues beauty as exemplified in slim and trim bodies. Many celebrities and stick-thin models present these products to us, and their sizes and shapes often add to the overall attraction of the products.

Some of the influences that affect your food choices can be positive, while others might not be so positive. Next time you see these influences coming on, stop and try to make a decision for yourself. Is that what you really wanted to eat, or did you just want to "fit in" with others? Ask yourself the following questions:

- Do you often agree to eat something just to go along with the crowd?
- Do others often make food decisions for you?
- Do you often buy something just because of an advertisement or television commercial, even if you know it's not the best choice?
- Do you tend to join friends for a meal, even if you don't care for the restaurant, just to be part of the group?
- Do you order foods you know your friends will like, just to have them like you better?

**FACTS**

**More than half of all food-related commercial advertisements are geared toward foods high in calories, fat, sugar, or salt.**

If you answered yes to two or more of these questions, then you need to become more aware of who is in control of your food decisions. Becoming aware of the influences that surround you is just one way you can begin to control your food intake and your overall health as well.

## Behaviors That Lead to Overeating

People, themselves, are guilty of eating for many reasons other than hunger. People eat because it's time to eat, because others are eating, or even because the food is there—it looks good and smells good. It's not uncommon for people to be labeled by the type of eater they are—a slow eater, fast eater, or a person who never eats sweets. Some people respond to environmental cues, such as an event or situation that triggers eating. The sight, smell, or familiar taste of a food can be a cue to stimulate eating. Social events, like parties, mealtimes, and watching television or going to the movies all serve as eating triggers, too.

**FACTS**

Frequent television watchers are more likely to feel "fatter" than their nonwatching counterparts, primarily due to the images that models and celebrities portray.

## Cravings

Cravings also lead a person to eat. A craving is defined as a strong desire to eat a particular food. Food cravings can occur any time of the day or night and are often affected by hormones, particularly in women, as observed during pregnancy and episodes of premenstrual syndrome. Dieters are also known to having frequent food cravings primarily because of their intense desire to eat a forbidden food.

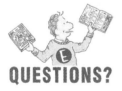

**QUESTIONS?**

**Do cravings really exist?**
A craving is described as a strong desire to eat a particular food, and yes, they do exist, many times in women who experience changes in hormone levels. Common cravings are for chocolate, ice cream, and sugary or fatty foods.

## Emotions

People use food in more ways than to just meet hunger and nourish the body. Many people express their emotions, like love or sorrow, with food. Food tends to make some people feel better. Others use food to fill an emotional void (as in the case of depression or loneliness). And still others offer food as a reward or punishment. In all cases, food becomes more than just nourishment for the body. A habitual attachment can grow as a result of reacting in the same manner to the same food stimulus over and over again.

# Physical Versus Emotional Hunger

Experts have now defined hunger in terms of physical hunger and emotional hunger. Physical hunger is defined as the state at which the body informs you of the need for food, as in a growling stomach. In contrast, emotional hunger is when a person eats to satisfy an emotional response, like a reaction to anxiety, loneliness, or stress.

Emotional hunger can become a problem for many people, but not all of us are prone to its effects. Emotional eating becomes a concern only when a person's responses to emotions become less and less controllable and when many different types of emotions can lead that person in the direction of food. Over time, these concerns can cause eating problems like obesity and food-related disorders like compulsive-eating disorder.

Food can bring on and satisfy many emotions—joy, excitement, anxiety, and even stress. People develop many emotional responses to food. Here are a few examples:

- As a child can you recall ever being given a treat to stop crying, or being promised an ice cream cone if you were good?
- Did your parents ever threaten to take away your dessert if you didn't eat your meal?
- Did boredom or loneliness ever send you in search of a snack in the refrigerator?
- Do you find yourself grabbing a cookie just after you've gotten upset or dishing out ice cream just because you are bored?
- Do you make popcorn just because you are going to watch a movie?
- Do you reach for certain foods referred to as "comfort foods," like macaroni and cheese, meat loaf, or mashed potatoes, because these bring you comfort?

Whenever you use food as a reliever of stress or anxiety, as a reward or punishment, to fill a void, or even to serve as an alternative to boredom or loneliness, you are placing a label on it and its importance to control emotional responses. You are sending a message that food can be tied to your behavior, whether for good reasons or bad.

So did you find some familiar behaviors within yourself? You can now begin to understand why you react to food the way you do.

## What Type of Eater Am I?

Do you find that environmental cues lead you to eat more frequently or that you have intense cravings for certain foods? Do you consider yourself a slow eater, a fast eater, an evening eater, a grazer, a member of the clean-the-plate club, or do you have your own label for the type of eater you are? Do you think you eat frequently as a result of stress or as a response to an argument with your boss or spouse?

Try to find out why and when you eat. Answer these questions:

- Do I eat even if I am not hungry?
- Do I eat just because others I am with are eating?
- Do I often eat so fast, I don't enjoy my food or know what I am eating?
- If something upsets me or causes me stress, do I seek out something to eat?
- Do I find myself looking for food when I am lonely or depressed?
- Do I often skip breakfast and lunch but make up for it later in the day?
- Do I clean my plate at every meal because I do not like waste?
- Do I pick food off of my children's plates when they don't finish it?

**E**SSENTIALS
You need to identify common behaviors, like eating in front of the television or snacking in the car, along with emotions like stress, anxiety, or frustration, that may trigger overeating.

Responding yes to any of these means you're using food in other ways than just to fill a need for hunger. Each and every one of us can be guilty of this behavior. We just need to be aware of the cues that cause us to eat and control them appropriately.

## Do I Eat Too Fast?

Sometimes it's hard to eat a meal with a slow eater if we tend to do the opposite and gulp our food down. Have you ever wondered why it takes a person so long to finish their meal or snack? These people really know how to enjoy their food. For those of us who are considered "fast eaters," we could learn a thing or two from our slow counterparts.

Eating fast can cause obesity. It can cause digestive problems. And, in many cases, fast eating results in our not tasting or enjoying our food or even knowing what we have just eaten. By eating food too fast, we eat more than we might even want or definitely more than we might need. It takes about twenty minutes from the time we begin eating to the time our stomach signals our brain that we might have had enough. If we continue to eat too fast, we tend to overfill our stomachs, thus causing possible indigestion and discomfort. This, too, pushes food through our digestive system too fast and may result in improper digestion. As a result, problems such as constipation, heartburn, or diarrhea may occur.

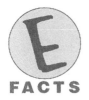

FACTS

Eat slow. It takes fifteen to twenty minutes for your stomach to signal your brain that it is full. Try soup, spicy foods, shellfish, artichokes—they take longer to eat.

As fast eaters we deny ourselves the opportunity to really enjoy our food. We all need to learn to sit back, relax, and take note from those slow eaters. You'll find yourself feeling full, feeling better, and maybe even having some leftovers for another meal.

## Am I a Grazer?

A grazer is a person who eats constantly, usually in small amounts and continually through the course of the day. This person never really has a chance to feel hunger. Children are often given this label when they continually ask for snacks and parents oblige. Their small stomachs are never empty enough to signal a hunger response. For adults, grazing develops out of boredom. Grazing is also a habit that frequent dieters can fall into, as they need to continue to feed their body without feeling signs of hunger.

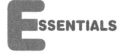

** SSENTIALS** The term *satiety* is used to explain the feeling of fullness one has after eating food. A sandwich that is higher in complex carbohydrates will provide a greater satiety value than a doughnut.

## Do I Starve All Day and Eat All Night?

Many people will admit to skipping breakfast, sometimes lunch, and only eating at dinnertime and bedtime. "Why am I so fat?" they say. "I don't eat all that much." Problems with this type of eating behavior stem from starving themselves to the point of extreme hunger and then eating more than is required in order to satisfy the hunger. When the body gets no food or fuel throughout the day, it begins to run down. At the point of physical hunger, almost anything and everything will look appetizing. Food will likely be consumed in more-than-adequate amounts. This is not a healthy behavior. The body cannot use food as efficiently when it's fed this way.

**ALERT** People who skip meals generally have a slower metabolism than those who do not because depriving the body of food causes its metabolism to slow down.

## Do I Belong to the Clean-the-Plate Club?

Years ago, our parents used to tell us to "clean our plate." We were told that kids all over the world were starving and that we shouldn't leave food on our plates. We were also told that food costs money, so we shouldn't throw it out. These comments have stuck with many people into adulthood. So, unconsciously, you might continue to clean your plate because you want to do no wrong. This can lead to problems with many individuals, because these plates may contain much more than you need to eat at one sitting.

It's not uncommon for parents with this kind of conditioning to also feel the need to clean their child's plate. We adults could learn a lot from our young children in that when they feel full, they walk away, often leaving food on their plates. Parents, in turn, need to walk away from this food too. There's no need to finish it off just to avoid throwing it out. Either learn to dish up smaller portions, or put it away for another time. What's the better choice—going to waste or going to waist?

## Tackling the Challenges of Overeating and Uncontrollable Overeating

So what can we do to avoid challenges with overeating? Here are some helpful tips to get you started:

- Don't skip meals. People of healthy weight typically eat three meals and one to two snacks each day. When you skip a meal, you set yourself up to overeat later.
- Eat meals and snacks in one place in your home (at the dining table). If you want to eat, you take the food to the table. Eating on the sofa, while watching television, or while you're walking throughout the house should be forbidden.
- Try to eat slower. Take your time. Talk to others at the table. Put your fork down once in a while. And learn to chew your food; learn to stop and enjoy its taste.
- Remove distractions. Turn off the television. Take away reading materials. Don't talk on the phone while eating. These all take your mind off of what you are eating and will cause you to eat more.
- Fill your plate at the stove, and put away the leftovers before you sit down to eat. This will keep you on target with eating allotted portions while helping you stay away from double servings just because it's there.

- Substitute other behaviors for eating. If you are stressed, talk a walk. If you are anxious, call a friend on the phone. If you are fidgety, start a project like knitting, needle pointing, painting, or compiling photographs into a scrapbook.
- Try to evaluate your need to eat and the cause of your eating. Keep a food diary like the one you'll find illustrated in the next section of this chapter. If you have difficulties identifying your problems, seek help from a registered dietitian.

## Starting a Diet Diary

Starting a diet diary is your first step in tackling some of the food-related behaviors that exist. Here you need to log the times you eat, your mood, hunger level, all of the foods eaten and how much of each food you eat. This diary is just a sample of the type that may help you. As you learn more about what and how you should be eating, you can put it all together to help conquer your problems once and for all. Another sample diet diary can be found in Chapter 19.

Time refers to the time at which you eat. Mood is how you feel. Are you happy, sad, frustrated, stressed, or nervous? These moods can all affect your eating decisions. Hunger Level refers to how hungry you are. Rate yourself from 1 to 5, 1 not being physically hungry at all and 5 being famished. Food Eaten is the food you selected and ate. Be specific. How Much indicates the portion size of the food you have selected. Again, be specific.

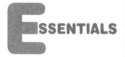

**ESSENTIALS** Seek out alternative behaviors to eating. Some options include taking a warm bath, joining a book club, making a fitness date, scheduling a massage, going to the movies, or even getting a haircut.

## SAMPLE DIET DIARY

| DAY 1 | TIME | MOOD | HUNGER LEVEL | FOOD EATEN | HOW MUCH |
|-------|------|------|--------------|------------|----------|
|       |      |      |              |            |          |
|       |      |      |              |            |          |
|       |      |      |              |            |          |

| DAY 2 | TIME | MOOD | HUNGER LEVEL | FOOD EATEN | HOW MUCH |
|-------|------|------|--------------|------------|----------|
|       |      |      |              |            |          |
|       |      |      |              |            |          |
|       |      |      |              |            |          |

| DAY 3 | TIME | MOOD | HUNGER LEVEL | FOOD EATEN | HOW MUCH |
|-------|------|------|--------------|------------|----------|
|       |      |      |              |            |          |
|       |      |      |              |            |          |

Now let's set a plan to make some changes. Remember, small changes can add to big results.

*This week I will try to*

*This month I will try to*

Determining why and what you eat is the key to understanding and managing changes in your overall lifestyle. Your behaviors reflect who you are. Behaviors are difficult to change. But just becoming aware of them can be the first major step in the right direction.

Start by using the sample diet diary illustrated here, or use the one found later in this book (in Chapter 19), for at least three to five days. Review your diary, or seek a professional to do so, and determine your problem areas and problem times during the day. Set some goals, short-term, to get yourself started and motivated. Take it one day at a time. As you begin to see positive results, you will likely feel better about yourself and what you can accomplish. Remember, you are doing this for you. Keep focused and keep motivated.

CHAPTER 4

# *How Fast Can I Lose?*

You are reading this because you have decided to lose some weight. You may want to take off as little as 10 pounds or maybe more than 50. And, you want to get those pounds off fast. You may not see the need to take the time to change habits and lifestyle patterns. You may feel it is not the time to think about health, about failing, and of course not about the cost. It's all worth it, right?

# The Current Diet Industry

Hundreds of diets are created and shared with us each and every year. We spend billions of dollars keeping the weight-loss industry alive—diets, gimmicks, beverages, powders, pills, equipment, and more. We find these every month in women's magazines, hear about them from friends, and see new celebrities promoting their new "diet" books and products through commercial advertisements and infomercials. Each diet claims to help you take off those extra pounds painlessly and effectively. Trends come and go, promising fast and easy weight-loss results. But if these diets really worked, would more and more come out each year? Would we always be looking for another one? Wouldn't we already be at our ideal weight?

## Weight-Loss Schemes

It's difficult for people to believe that our world can be so scientifically and technologically advanced and yet that medical miracles in weight loss just don't exist. We all wish dieting could be miracle-easy, but unfortunately it is not. Losing weight is just one of those processes that cannot be controlled through a quick process. As much as we want to believe what we hear, an immediate red flag should go up if you see promotions like these:

- Easy and effortless
- Guaranteed to work
- Miracle results
- Miraculous
- Breakthrough
- New discovery
- Fast working
- Magic pill, magic formula, or magical cure
- Quick weight loss
- Secret formula
- Eat one type of food only
- Eat food in a particular order

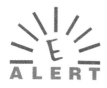

Anyone can make a claim about losing weight. Anyone can sell a diet. Anyone can promote a weight-loss product. Beware of fraudulent moneymaking schemes.

## Diet Success Stories

Of course we are inspired by those fabulous success stories and promises like "Drop 10 pounds in a week," "Shrink your stomach," or "Lose two dress sizes in one month." And those remarkable before and after pictures. Are these really the same person? Why wouldn't we be intrigued? It sounds so good. But that may be just it—too good to be true.

# The Real Story of Fad Dieting

First and foremost, you need to accept the fact that losing weight healthfully and effectively is not effortless. It requires much planning, insight, and motivation. Fad dieting, on the other hand, is just that—a fad. Fad diets are trendy. They do not stay around for any length of time. They also can be risky and dangerous, and they rarely provide long-term, effective results.

## Your Desire to Lose—Quick and Painlessly

Is it really so important that this weight come off today and now? Let's begin by looking at why you are desperate to lose:

- Are you so obsessed with the idea of losing weight that you would sacrifice your overall health?
- Do you often compare your size to that of another person?
- Do you think being obese makes you lazy, sloppy, and undisciplined?
- Do you believe that losing weight will make you well liked and popular among your friends?
- Do you insist on crash dieting before any big social gathering?

Responding positively to any of these questions puts you in the category for being obsessed with your weight. It happens to many of us.

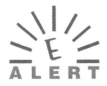

Stay clear of fad diets, crash diets, and fasting diets. They may reduce your weight, but they can also result in serious side effects and health complications. These diets rarely lead to permanent results because the radical changes they bring about are difficult to maintain over long periods of time.

## Trying Anything and Everything

We know we want the excess pounds to go away badly—so badly that we will do anything to get them off. We will try any diet, drink any concoction, and seek any weight-loss recommendations—whatever is "hot" at the time—without any knowledge of what we are doing to ourselves. What we notice over time is that these diets do work initially. A few pounds do come off. But soon enough they return. And then next month or next year we are back where we started. The process begins again and again. Sometimes we are even worse off than where we started. Where do we go from here?

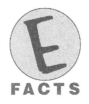

More than 90 percent of dieters who lose weight tend to regain it all (and sometimes more) within five years. That makes only a small 5 to 10 percent of all dieters who are successful enough to keep it off for five years or more.

## The All-Dreaded Diet

The word *diet* means "manner of living," originally meant to encompass an entire approach to eating and daily activities. Today, the term dieting can be confusing to many people. Although the term *diet* can refer to any eating pattern, it is primarily used to describe a plan of restricted eating that may include some, if any, nutritional guidance. Many of these restricted or deprived eating patterns are not a healthy option for anyone.

In fact, even though hundreds of diets are released each year, many of the same people try these new diets again and again.

Don't get me wrong, weight will be lost on these restricted diets. That is a fact. But is it the healthiest way to lose? No. Will the weight likely come back again? You bet. Most weight lost on severely restricted diets is usually regained within a year of its loss. Somewhere in the neighborhood of only 5 to 10 percent of people actually keep their weight off for more than five years when it is lost through restrictive diets. And for the majority of people, the original pounds plus more are put back on.

**FACTS**

The word *diet* comes from the Greek word *diaita*, which means "manner of living." Scientists and researchers agree that one's diet and daily activities encompass an entire "manner of living" and not a pattern of restricted eating.

## Dieting as a Temporary State

The decision to diet is dreaded by most people. The word *diet* is often referred to as a "four-letter word." The state of dieting can be a chore. Dieting is usually viewed as a temporary situation to be tolerated until the desired results are reached. Then it often becomes forgotten. Old eating habits return, and the body returns to its original shape and size. Dieting is an unpleasant task. It can be expensive and is generally unhealthy. Yo-yo dieting becomes a common result. Yo-yo dieting refers to the continuous cycle of going on and off diets, losing and regaining the weight. By doing so, a person's metabolism is constantly being changed. This results in possible medical complications while doing havoc to one's self-esteem at the same time. Dieting as a result becomes counterproductive and potentially harmful.

## The Problem with Improper Dieting

Of course, there are many restrictive eating plans that indeed do the job, but there are many more that do not. Some can be extremely harmful, too, if adhered to for extended periods of time. Some diets stress particular foods others insist you eat foods in a special order. Some programs are "right for your type," while others require medical supervision. Some put unrealistic expectations on caloric levels, and still others may be all liquid, no solid foods. The Food and Drug Administration does not check out all these programs before they are released; in fact, many come from clever merchandisers who know how to attract consumers. Here is the problem with improper dieting:

- Quick weight-loss diets don't work for the long haul. Losing weight quickly deprives your body of the food it needs to survive and likely results in not loss of extra body fat, but actually of body water and muscle.
- Dieting slows down metabolism. In a severe dieting state, your body thinks it is starving. It goes into a starvation mode to conserve extra energy and store fat, therefore slowing overall metabolism.
- Dieting can be expensive. Desperate people will spend whatever it takes when they're seeking results, including pills, powders, gadgets, equipment, and books that can add up the dollars and cents.
- Dieting doesn't necessarily make you healthier or more fit. Being thin isn't always about being healthier or being more fit, because skinny people can be just as "out of shape" and unhealthy as overweight people.
- Dieting can actually cause weight gain. Severely restricted diets might help you lose weight and fast, but once old eating habits return, pounds usually do, too, putting the weight back on and oftentimes more.
- Dieting can lower self-esteem. Isn't it embarrassing to drop 20 pounds and show it off, then regain 40 pounds?
- Dieting can cause irritability and mood changes. Over time, dieters can often develop mood swings due to the types of food (and nutrients) they omit from their diet.
- Dieting can be harmful. Eating unbalanced proportions of the energy-contributing nutrients (protein, carbohydrates, and fat) can often be harmful to normal body functions.

**FACTS**

Dieting by eating an abundance of foods that primarily include diet soft drinks, fat-free/no-fat, and low-fat products deprives the body of its required nutrient needs.

## What Happens When We Diet Improperly?

Depending on the particular process we follow in restricting food intake, many things can happen. Here are just a few to note:

| WHEN WE . . . | HOW WE RESPOND . . . |
|---|---|
| **Skip meals** | • The body's need for fuel and energy causes extreme hunger.<br>• Metabolism is lowered.<br>• Eating can be excessive and uncontrollable.<br>• More quantities of food will likely be consumed overall. |
| **Eat very few calories (fewer than 800 per day)** | • Primarily lose water and muscle weight.<br>• Our metabolism is lowered.<br>• Get moody and tired.<br>• Heartbeat can become irregular.<br>• The body can go into a state of ketosis (a condition where the body uses other sources of energy when carbohydrates are not available, leading to dangerous consequences). |
| **Fast** | • The body is deprived of energy and fuel from necessary nutrients.<br>• We may become fatigued and dizzy.<br>• We lose water and muscle weight.<br>• Our metabolism is lowered. |
| **Eat only high-protein foods** | • We feel moody, tired, and have little energy from not eating carbohydrates, our primary energy source.<br>• Can lead to nausea, dehydration, constipation, headaches, and loss of muscle tissue. |

| WHEN WE . . . | HOW WE RESPOND . . .  (continued) |
|---|---|
| **Eat only high-protein foods** | • We tend to consume too many high-fat, high-cholesterol, and high-calorie foods that can increase risk of heart disease and possibly some types of cancers.<br>• Our diet can lack essential vitamins/minerals/complex carbohydrates/fiber.<br>• Too much protein may remove calcium from the bones.<br>• The body can go into a state of ketosis (a condition where the body uses other sources of energy when carbohydrates are not available, leading to dangerous health consequences.) |
| **Eat only high-carb foods** | • We can become fatigued.<br>• We tend to consume a high concentration of fiber, which can lead to constipation and dehydration.<br>• Can result in hair loss or weak fingernails. |
| **Consume liquid-diet formulas for all meals** | • Weight loss results mostly from water, body fluids, and muscle weight.<br>• Can result in irregular heartbeats.<br>• Our metabolism is lowered.<br>• Results can lead to fatigue, kidney problems, dehydration, nausea, constipation, diarrhea, loss of hair.<br>• We don't learn how to eat properly. |
| **Consume liquid-diet formulas for one meal per day** | • Weight loss results from water and muscle weight.<br>• Diet could be low in protein/carbohydrates/vitamins/minerals.<br>• We learn to rely too heavily on formulas, not foods. |
| **Follow trendy/novelty programs** | • Food choices lack variety and can be unbalanced.<br>• Diet is usually low in protein, vitamins, and minerals.<br>• Can result in dizziness, diarrhea, hair loss, weak fingernails, loss of muscle tissue. |

# Psychological Concerns from Excess Dieting

People who try new diets frequently spend a great deal of time and energy worrying about food, especially what they will eat next and what they can't cat at all. On almost every program, the challenge is to follow the eating plan rules, but the number of people who comply and actually stay on them is low. This causes extreme anxiety, especially if (and when) failure results (at least according to the number illustrated on the bathroom scale). To compensate for a lack of success, dieting may also lead to excessive overeating, undereating, depression, and guilt feelings toward food.

Mixed messages from the media and friends about the "hot diet that worked for me" draws people in droves to try the next trendy plan. If failures continue, inadequacies about one's ability to succeed increases. These failures compound and can cause psychological problems along with the physical problems.

## Spotting a Fad Diet

Fad diets are categorized as those that promote quick weight loss. In many cases, these diets are restrictive, unbalanced, offer unrealistic promises and can lead to health and related problems. Weight will be lost, initially, but most likely it will be regained. And on top of it all, results are usually temporary at best, so frustration follows. People who choose to follow these diets often feel like failures because they cannot stick with them.

Any and all of these common denominators can be found in fad diets:

- These diets are essentially low or very low in calories and although not advertised as such, are usually well below caloric recommendations.
- These diets are deficient in many nutrients, including carbohydrates and fiber, and many vitamins and minerals.
- These diets are well out of balance of dietary recommendations, requiring too many proteins and fats and too few carbohydrates or too many carbohydrates and too little protein and fat.
- These diets cause initial weight loss from body fluids, thus giving dieters a sense of accomplishment, when in fact the weight will soon return, and accomplishments will turn into failures.
- These diets do not promote portion size. They do not teach consumers how to eat in moderation.

- Some of these diets encourage "food combining," eating certain foods together or apart.
- Many recommend that dieters follow suggested eating plans for extended periods of time.
- Often these diets discourage long-term compliance, knowing how harmful they may be if followed for extended periods of time.

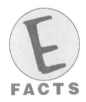

**FACTS**

Portion size is rarely addressed in a fad diet. The focus is primarily on eliminating an entire food category rather than just eating less of it.

The initial thought of a quick fad diet is encouraging to many people—just lose a quick 5 to 10 pounds. But long-term consequences are much greater. Fad diets just don't work. Don't start a habit of being drawn in to these programs. You will just set yourself up for disappointment that will ultimately make you feel like you have failed. Seek better choices for yourself. Gradual changes that require long-term modifications to your eating patterns and lifestyle make more sense all the way around. If you are really willing to try anything to lose the weight, why not do it the right way?

## What about Weight-Loss Medications?

Weight-loss medications have recently become a popular trend in our country. All of us would agree that taking a pill that would encourage weight loss is the ideal. Who wouldn't want to try it?

Even if you want to believe that this is the newest trend in weight loss, people have been taking medications for years in hopes of dropping weight. The old "diet pills" that doctors used to give out some forty to fifty years ago primarily contained amphetamines, were highly addictive, and led to adverse effects on the heart and nervous system. These compounds are no longer recommended for use in obesity treatment. Other medications we might be familiar with are easily purchased over the counter at the drugstore and are mostly known to decrease the appetite.

While the FDA regulates how a medication can be advertised or promoted, no one can regulate a doctor's ability to properly prescribe it.

## Common Side Effects

Common side effects of weight-loss medications may include the following:

- Irregular heartbeat
- High blood pressure
- Anxiety
- Headaches
- Seizures
- Heart attack/stroke
- High cholesterol
- Fatigue/tiredness
- Weakness/fainting/dizziness
- Gallstones
- Anemia/low iron levels
- Nausea
- Death

Diet drugs and medications are not intended for overweight and marginally obese people. The harmful effects of long-term use of these drugs and medications can outweigh the health benefits of losing weight.

## Recent Medication Developments

In recent years, various medications have been released to the public to help lose extreme amounts of weight. These products were promoted as a new type of appetite suppressant. Over the period of several years, millions of prescriptions were written, primarily to overweight women seeking quick weight-loss results.

Various side effects and health concerns associated with some medications later caused them to be removed from the market. But due to consumer interest in such products, the market was wide open for new medications. As a result, manufacturers, weight-loss professionals, and others began promoting and releasing new prescription, over-the-counter, and herbal remedies to promote weight loss.

Although many more new products have since been released, and although people are more skeptical of product safety, there is still no lack of consumer interest in purchasing new options. People continue to line up to try the latest medication in hopes of dropping those extra, unnecessary pounds.

Products like appetite suppressants used to decrease appetite and increase satiety (the feeling of fullness) and products used to block absorption of fat and even starches can be found in abundance. But none of these products is marketed to work alone. People forget that along with taking these "pills," instructions also state the importance of making lifestyle changes by decreasing total food intake and increasing activity levels. Maybe this helps some people get started, maybe not.

Primarily prescription medications were promoted to the severely obese. Even with their so-called side effects, these medications were believed by experts to be less of a health risk than being seriously obese. As time went on, more and more prescriptions were being written for cosmetic reasons and for many people who were less than severely obese. People need to realize that these drugs are powerful. They can be harmful if not used properly.

**ALERT**

Appetite-suppressant medications can be harmful and should be used only by patients who are at increased risk of medical problems because of obesity and not for cosmetic reasons to lose weight.

With use of these medications, pounds will be lost. But pounds will stay off only as long as the plan is continued. Once medications stop and old lifestyle habits return, pounds are regained. Medications serve again as only a temporary solution.

## Weight-Loss Medication Schemes

Beware of the following weight-loss medications and products. The Food and Drug Administration has banned many of these products since they've hit the market.

- Pills claiming to "burn fat": These products include such ingredients as alcohol, caffeine, dextrose, and guar gum and claimed to dissolve excess fat.
- "Diet patches": These are promoted as a means to dispatch medication through a patch placed on the skin.
- "Fat blockers": These promote the blockage of fat absorption.
- "Starch blockers": These promote the blockage of starch absorption.
- "Bulk fillers": These include excess fiber to fill the stomach and absorb fluids.
- "Magnet-type" pills: These are promoted as a way to flush out the body.

## Herbal Remedies

Recent trends and interest have also led to a large market of herbal remedies designed to help a person lose weight. These natural products are available through health food stores, mall kiosks, Internet sales, weight-loss clinics, individual distributors, and drug stores. The Food and Drug Administration warns consumers about the harmful use of many of these products, as their safety and effectiveness have not been tested.

Many herbal products contain an amphetamine-like compound with potentially harmful stimulant effects on the heart and central nervous system. Some of these products act as diuretics (substances that increase urine production), thus causing water weight loss. Others are promoted to increase metabolism and decrease appetite. Products like these often can lead to undesirable side effects like insomnia, irregular heartbeats, tremors, headaches, irritability, and high blood pressure. There are still other products that offer the benefit of helping consumers feel satiated or full. These products tend to absorb fluids in the body, make a person feel fuller, but in reality they have little weight-loss benefit.

## Weight-Loss Effects from Hot and Spicy Foods

Hot and spicy foods often are promoted as foods and spices that can help increase your metabolism (the rate at which calories are burned). Reports indicate that these foods do not increase your metabolism, but may just increase your desire to consume liquids because of their hot, spicy flavors.

Herbs, over-the-counter medications, and prescription medications are all drugs with potential side effects. Some are tested for their safety, but long-term studies take time. Testing each and every one of them is not possible. Consumers need to be cautious of products they take and be more aware of possible health consequences that may result.

# Surgery as a Weight-Loss Option

Some individuals have even sought out surgery as an extreme weight-loss option. This process limits the amount of food that can move into the stomach by closing off or removing parts of the stomach or by causing food to bypass the stomach or part of the intestine during digestion. This extreme weight-loss option is primarily used for individuals 100 or more pounds overweight. It is usually provided as a result of other health complications that may be occurring. Consumers need to understand that this option carries many health risks as well.

Have you found the ultimate diet of your dreams? None of the programs or products discussed in this chapter is the dream diet. You need to be the judge over what you do to your body and what works for you. Don't be taken in by overzealous claims. Don't throw away your good sense of nutrition or your need to establish lifelong healthy habits. Balance your food choices and eat a variety of foods, doing so in moderation. Restrictive dieting results in overall ineffective weight loss and management. The expectation of temporary changes leading to long-term results is not the way to go. Learn to be realistic. Learn to be sensible. In the next few chapters you will find some alternative, healthier options to meet your weight-loss needs.

CHAPTER 5

# Dietary Guidelines
# for Americans

The study of nutrition and the foods we eat can be confusing and often tricky for those of us not trained in this area. But it isn't necessary to have a degree in nutrition to understand and practice nutrition guidelines that promote health and prevent the onset of disease.

## Current Guidelines

Back in the early 1980s, the United States Department of Agriculture, along with the Department of Health and Human Services, created the first Dietary Guidelines for Americans as a means of helping people understand what they should be eating to stay healthy. People of various cultural backgrounds, age groups, and lifestyles should be able to follow these basic guidelines. But they need to realize that these are just guidelines—suggestions to help people stay healthy. These guidelines are written to apply to the healthy American population over two years of age and are updated every five years to supply consumers with the most current nutrition information available.

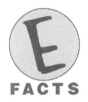

**FACTS**

All adults should strive for at least thirty minutes of moderate physical activity each day. Moderate activity is any activity that uses as much energy as walking two miles in thirty minutes.

The latest dietary guidelines were updated in 2000. They were written to provide simple, consistent messages to help consumers achieve and maintain healthy, active lifestyles. Flexibility is offered to help consumers make the best food choices for themselves.

Three basic messages can be found within these new guidelines. These include:

- **A:** Aim for fitness.
- **B:** Build a healthy base.
- **C:** Choose sensibly.

## Aim for Fitness

The two parts of aiming for fitness are aiming for a healthy weight and being physically active each day.

## Seek and Maintain a Healthy Weight

Seeking and maintaining a healthy weight is key to obtaining health. As discussed in Chapter 2, every individual should evaluate their weight to determine risk for obesity and other chronic diseases. Although many options for determining healthy weight are available, the most popular, accessible, and easiest to use is the Body Mass Index (BMI). This tool uses a mathematical formula to determine the ratio between a person's height and weight. BMI measurements are far from perfect, but they do provide a general guideline for determining healthy weight. To determine your own BMI, see Chapter 2 (page 23).

## Be Physically Active Each Day

One important way to achieve and maintain a healthy lifestyle is to incorporate physical activity into your day along with a daily sensible eating plan. This will also help you to achieve a healthy weight. By doing so, you will avoid gaining excess body weight that can over time increase health risks such as heart disease, high blood pressure, diabetes, stroke, arthritis, and certain types of cancers. In the meantime, learn to improve and increase your physical activity. Being more active allows you to burn extra calories and energy.

**E**SSENTIALS — Food made from sources of grains (wheat, rice, and oats) form the foundation of a healthy, nutritious diet.

Instead of sitting around watching television or working on the computer, join a fitness club, play tennis, ride bikes, or just take a walk. And, remember, no one is too old or too young to reap the benefits of regular physical activity. More can be found on the benefits of exercise in Chapter 14.

## Build a Healthy Base

Building a healthy base is comprised of letting the Food Guide Pyramid guide your food choices; choosing a variety of grains daily, especially whole grains; choosing a variety of fruits and vegetables daily; and keeping food safe to eat.

## Let the Pyramid Guide Your Food Choices

Because no one single food can provide all the nutrients you need, you should consume a number of different foods each day. The Food Guide Pyramid (outlined in Chapter 6) is a tool that helps you do just this by helping you to balance food choices, to select a variety of different foods, and to eat foods in moderate portions. This pyramid helps put the Dietary Guidelines for Americans into practice by emphasizing the importance of eating a combination of whole grains, fruits and vegetables, lower-fat dairy products, and lean meats daily.

## Choose a Variety of Grains Daily

Foods that are made from grains (wheat, rice, and oats) form the basis for a healthy diet. In addition to supplying a vast collection of vitamins and minerals, these foods add fiber and other essential nutrients to the diet. Grain products are also typically low in fat, unless fat is added during preparation or when served at the table.

## Choose a Variety of Fruits and Vegetables Daily

Eating a variety of fruits and vegetables in addition to grains each day is the best way to get started on a plan for healthier eating. Here you can begin to incorporate complex carbohydrates into the diet. Complex carbohydrates or foods that are primarily high in starch and dietary fiber add great nutrition benefits to the diet. Dietary fiber, sometimes called *roughage*, is not a nutrient as such, but refers to the substances in food that resist digestion. The amount of fiber in a food is based on the type of plant source it originated from and also depending on how it was processed. Highly processed foods offer less fiber than those that are less processed.

There are two distinct types of fiber: soluble fiber and insoluble fiber. Plant foods often contain a mixture of both types. Soluble fiber forms a gel-like substance in water and will dissolve or bulk up in hot water. Foods containing soluble fiber are fruits, vegetables, and grains, including prunes, pears, apples, oranges, legumes, dried beans and peas, sweet potatoes, cauliflower, zucchini, brown rice, oat, and corn bran. These foods tend to add bulk and thickness to the contents in the stomach upon digestion, thus making a person feel more full and satisfied after eating them.

Dieters often are encouraged to consume many sources of these fibrous foods because these foods tend to fill up a person up more quickly and decrease appetite, thus resulting in less food eaten overall. Soluble fiber is also known to lower blood cholesterol levels and improve blood glucose levels of individuals with diabetes.

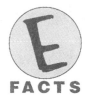

**FACTS**

Fiber acts like a sponge by absorbing water that softens stools and reduces incidence of constipation. Fiber is helpful in weight management and reduction in that it helps provide a sensation of fullness by actually slowing the emptying time of the stomach. Fibrous foods are also usually low in fat and calories.

Insoluble fiber, on the other hand, does not dissolve in water although it does add bulk to the intestinal content during digestion. In doing so, foods with insoluble fiber speed up the time it takes foods to travel through the intestine. Consumption of insoluble fiber helps in preventing constipation, problems with hemorrhoids, and a condition called *diverticular disease*. In addition, a high-fiber diet may also reduce the risk of colon cancer. Our best source of insoluble fiber comes from wheat bran. Other sources include whole grains, dried beans and peas, and most fruits and vegetables (and particularly their skin).

A high-fiber diet can be beneficial in health as well as in weight reduction. Here's how you can build up your fiber intake:

- Choose whole-grain breads instead of white.
- Choose whole-grain and bran cereals.
- Use brown rice over white rice. Also try other whole-wheat grain products.
- Snack on popcorn.

- Add fresh vegetables like lettuce, tomato, onions, and cucumbers to your sandwich.
- Snack on whole fresh fruit, eating the skin. Also eat the skin of your baked potato.
- Top salads with crunchy toppings like garbanzo beans, nuts, and seeds.
- Try bean and vegetable soups.

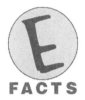

**FACTS**

Dietary fiber is lacking in many American diets. Daily recommendations suggest consuming an intake of 20 to 35 grams of fiber. Most Americans get only about half of that amount on a daily basis, if that much.

Along with contributing fiber, fruits and vegetables contribute different nutrients to the diet as well. Some may be excellent sources of vitamin A, like dark green leafy lettuce, whereas others may be high in vitamin C, like oranges and other citrus fruits. Most fruits and vegetables also offer the benefit of being low in fat and high in fiber. Your best shot at consuming the required amount of fruits and vegetables each day would be to aim for five a day—five total servings.

Try these creative suggestions for upping your intake.

- Top cereals or yogurt with berries or sliced fruit.
- Grate carrots or zucchini and add them to casseroles, quick breads, rice, and pasta dishes.
- Spread pizzas with a variety of vegetables.
- Try different types of fruit and vegetable juices (cranberry, papaya, mango, tomato).
- Substitute half of the margarine in homemade bread, muffin, and cookie recipes with applesauce, mashed bananas, or puréed prunes.
- Add extra toppings (shredded carrots or zucchini, sliced cucumbers or tomatoes) to sandwiches.
- Make stir-fry meals.
- Pack fresh and dried fruit for car trips.

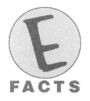

**FACTS**

Experts agree that a dietary intake high in vegetables, fruits, whole grains, dried beans and peas, and that is low in fat is essential in avoiding risk of chronic conditions and diseases like heart disease, stroke, and certain types of cancers.

## Keep Food Safe to Eat

**FIGURE 5-1:** Safe cooking temperatures

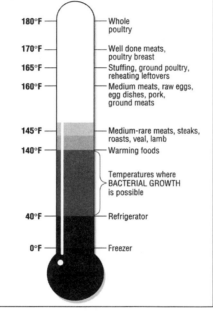

Whatever types of foods you choose to eat, make sure you keep them safe. Safe foods mean that the food is wholesome and free from harmful bacteria, viruses, parasites, and chemical contaminants. Food manufacturers, growers, producers, and supermarkets are responsible for making your foods as safe as possible at the time of purchasing. You are responsible for practicing food safety in your home and away to ensure that you are eating the safest foods you can.

Here are several ways you can make your foods as safe as they can be:

- Wash your hands often when preparing and serving foods.
- Wash raw fruits and vegetables before eating.
- Clean countertops, surfaces, sinks, and sponges regularly.
- Keep raw meats away from cooked ones.
- Thaw frozen meat in the refrigerator, under cool running water, or in a microwave oven, not on a countertop at room temperature.
- Always cook foods to safe temperatures.
- Serve hot foods hot (at or above 140°F) and cold foods cold (at or below 40°F).
- Chill leftovers soon after eating, and use them within three to four days.
- Don't eat any food that is questionable. If you are unsure of its safety, throw it out.

Temperatures of 60° to 125°F encourage rapid bacteria growth. Cooked foods should never stay at these temperatures for more than two hours.

The best way to determine whether meat, poultry, and egg dishes are cooked properly and safely is to use a food thermometer to test their internal temperatures. A thermometer, available at many stores, will allow you to ensure your food is cooked thoroughly and safe to eat.

# Choose Sensibly

Choosing sensibly means choosing a diet that is low in saturated fat and cholesterol and moderate in total fat; choosing beverages and foods to moderate your intake of sugars; choosing and preparing foods with less salt; and only drinking alcoholic beverages in moderation.

## Choose a Diet Low in Saturated Fat and Cholesterol

You may be surprised to know that we do need to eat fat in the diet. Fats supply essential fatty acids and help absorb fat-soluble vitamins (vitamins A, D, E, and K) in the body. But problems arise because people tend to eat too much fat.

Diets high in fat, particularly saturated fat and cholesterol, both known to increase blood cholesterol levels, have been linked to heart disease, stroke, obesity, and certain types of cancer. In contrast, consuming fats from unsaturated sources (mainly from vegetable oils) does not raise blood cholesterol levels. Eating too much fat, of all types, is also a cause of obesity.

Because of the concern with high-fat foods and a high-fat diet, recommendations call for choosing a diet with no greater than 30 percent of the total calories coming from fat. Of this 30 percent, no more than 10 percent should come from saturated fat sources. Refer to the following chart to see how many grams of fat, saturated and unsaturated, should be part of a diet depending on the number of calories consumed daily.

| DAILY CALORIES | TOTAL GRAMS OF FAT (30%) | TOTAL CALORIES FROM FAT (9/GRAM) | GRAMS OF SATURATED FAT (10%) | CALORIES FROM SATURATED FAT (30% OF TOTAL SATURATED FAT) |
|---|---|---|---|---|
| 1,200 | 40 | 360 | 13 | 117 |
| 1,500 | 50 | 450 | 17 | 153 |
| 1,800 | 60 | 540 | 20 | 180 |
| 2,000 | 67 | 600 | 22 | 198 |
| 2,500 | 83 | 747 | 28 | 252 |

Saturated fats are primarily found in foods from animal sources, like high-fat dairy products (whole milk and cheese), fatty fresh and processed meats, skin and fat on poultry, lard, and also in palm and coconut oils. Cholesterol is also found solely in animal products, primarily in the liver and other organ meats, egg yolks, dairy fats, chicken skin, fatty meats, and in some seafood. Unsaturated fats are mainly found in vegetable oils, nuts, olives, avocados, and fatty fish like salmon. All are considered fats. Some are healthier choices than others but in all cases their intake should be limited.

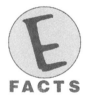

**FACTS**

Recommendations call for individuals to consume less than 300 milligrams of cholesterol per day.

In order to follow these recommendations, here's how you can reduce your fat and cholesterol intake:

- Reduce the amount of fat you consume from animal sources, like fat on meats and fat in milk, butter, cream, and egg yolks.
- Choose lean cuts of meat.
- Remove skin from chicken and poultry before eating.
- Select low-fat dairy products, including milk, yogurt, cheese, and cottage cheese.
- Limit your intake of high-fat convenience snack foods.
- Limit foods like cookies, cakes, pastries, doughnuts, margarine, and cooking oils.

- Become familiar with sources of saturated fat and cholesterol.
- Use low-fat soft margarine in place of hard margarine.
- Use liquid cooking spray in place of oil or butter.
- Avoid fried foods; opt for baked, broiled, boiled, or grilled foods instead.
- Substitute olive oil, canola oil, or other vegetable oils for solid fats like margarine, butter, or lard.
- Be smart, too, and compare similar products.

Be a wise shopper. Know what you are buying and what you are eating. So many similar-seeming products are really not that similar at all in nutrient content. Be sure to read the labels so you really understand what is in the product you choose. Here are several comparisons.

| FOOD | AMOUNT | SATURATED FAT (GRAMS) | CHOLESTEROL (MG) |
| --- | --- | --- | --- |
| Cheddar cheese | 1 ounce | 6 | 30 |
| Low-fat Cheddar cheese | 1 ounce | 1.2 | 6 |
| Fat-free Cheddar cheese | 1 ounce | 0 | 3 |
| Whole milk | 1 cup | 5.1 | 33.2 |
| 2% milk | 1 cup | 3 | 20 |
| Skim milk | 1 cup | .4 | 5 |
| Croissant | 1 | 6.6 | 33.2 |
| Plain bagel | 1 | .16 | 0 |
| Ice cream | ½ cup | 7.4 | 45.1 |
| Sherbet | ½ cup | 1.1 | 5.9 |
| Frozen yogurt | ½ cup | .8 | 5.1 |
| Butter | 1 tsp. | 2.4 | 10.4 |
| Margarine | 1 tsp. | .65 | 0 |
| Imitation margarine | 1 tsp. | .3 | 0 |

*Product values from different manufacturers may differ slightly.

Foods high in saturated fats tend to raise blood cholesterol levels. These are found primarily in foods from animal origin. Dietary cholesterol also can raise blood cholesterol levels and is found in foods of animal origin as well. Unsaturated fats do not raise blood cholesterol levels and are found primarily in vegetable sources. Although a wiser choice, these are still 100 percent fat.

## Moderate Your Intake of Sugar

Limiting your intake of sugar will likely help control your total calorie intake, decrease the incidence of obesity, and reduce risk of tooth decay. Sugars can be found in table sugar (sucrose) or in the form of complex sugars like fructose (sugar found in fruit and honey) and lactose (sugar found in milk).

Your body cannot tell the difference between simple or complex sugars or sugars that come from natural or refined sources—all are broken down into glucose during digestion to provide a quick source of energy. Foods high in sugar include white table sugar, brown sugar, honey, molasses, jellies, table syrups, soft drinks, fruit drinks, flavored beverages, candies, and dessert foods. Many of these foods are referred to as "empty calorie" foods as they offer calories but very few nutrients. People often consume excess sugary foods in place of more nutritious choices. Other foods like potatoes and orange juice also contain sugar but provide other valuable nutrients as well, so these types of foods would not be considered empty-calorie foods. Wouldn't you think an apple would be a better choice as a snack than a candy bar? Or how about a glass of orange juice over a soft drink?

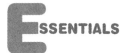

There is no benefit to using honey over sugar. Your body cannot distinguish between table sugar and the complex sugars found in honey, fruit, or milk. It cannot tell whether sugar comes from a natural or refined source. All forms of sugar are broken down during digestion into glucose for energy.

The USDA recommends limiting added sugars in the diet to 6 to 10 percent of total daily calories. (Each teaspoon of sugar equals about 16 calories.) If you eat 1,200 calories per day, that equals no more than 72 to 120 calories from sugar, or 4½ to 7½ teaspoons; if you eat 1,600 calories per day, that means no more than 96 to 160 calories from sugar, or 6 to 10 teaspoons per day; and if you eat 2,200 calories per day, that means no more than 132 to 220 calories from sugar, or 8 to 14 teaspoons.

Sugar is found in many obvious food choices, like candies, cookies, cakes, and pastries, but also it can be found in many not-so-obvious food choices, like milk, breads, and fruits. But keep in mind that the foods that contain sugar (those empty-calorie foods) and no other nutrition are the ones with which you need to be concerned.

| Food Source | Amount | Teaspoons of Sugar |
| --- | --- | --- |
| Premium cheesecake | 1 slice | 12 |
| Fruit-flavored beverage | ¾ cup | 6 |
| Iced cupcake or slice of cake | 1 | 5 |
| Glazed doughnut | 1 | 4 |
| Ice cream | ½ cup | 4 |
| Chocolate-covered ice cream bar | 1 | 3½ |
| Chocolate-filled sandwich cookies | 3 | 3½ |
| Jelly | 1 Tbsp. | 3 |
| Presweetened cereal | 1 cup | 3 |
| Fruit leather roll | 1 | 2½ |

Now, look at some of your favorite foods to see how many teaspoons of sugar they contain. To do so, look at the Nutrition Facts Label, find the grams of sugar, and divide this number by four. In the case of a 12-ounce can of soft drink, we find it has 41 grams of sugar. Divided by four, that equals 10 teaspoons. Wow!

Don't be fooled by other names commonly used in place of sugar on product labels. These include products like the following.

- Brown sugar
- Cane sugar
- Confectioner's (powdered) sugar
- Corn syrup
- Corn sweeteners
- Dextrin
- Dextrose
- Fruit juice concentrate
- Fructose
- High-fructose corn syrup
- Honey
- Glucose
- Granulated sugar
- Invert sugar
- Lactose
- Malt syrup
- Maple sugar
- Maltose
- Molasses
- Raw sugar
- Sucrose
- Turbinado sugar

Sugar is an important component of anyone's diet, but it does need to be consumed in moderation. Here are several suggestions for how you can control your intake of overall sugar:

- Limit beverages that add excess sugar to your diet.
- Watch nutrition labels for hidden forms of sugar.
- Limit "empty calorie" foods, like candies, cookies, pies, cakes, and pastries that contribute sugar and little else.
- Learn to enjoy the taste of foods without added sugar, as in the case of cereal, tea, and coffee.

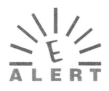

Soft drinks are the number one contributor of sugar in the American diet. A 12-ounce can of regular soft drink contributes 10 teaspoons of sugar alone.

## Choose and Prepare Foods with Less Salt

You may or may not be instructed to reduce your overall salt intake in your diet, but it is a good idea for all people to limit salt (or sodium) intake. Too much salt in the diet, is linked with high blood pressure. Many foods add salt to the diet, including processed foods, soups, luncheon meats, snack foods, and beverages.

Sodium is important to the body in regulating fluids and blood pressure. Too much sodium in the diet can also cause a person to retain fluids and as a result increase the numbers on the scale due to an increase in water weight.

Since there are not indicators for who will develop high blood pressure from consuming excess salt, recommendations for daily sodium intake should be no more than 2,400 milligrams per day. This is about the amount of salt found in one teaspoon.

Salt, or sodium chloride, is the primary source of sodium found in foods. There is little naturally occurring salt in the foods we eat. Most salt is added during processing or through use of the saltshaker during food preparation or at the table. Your best attempt in reducing sodium intake is to do away with the extra use of salt at home and away.

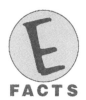

**FACTS**

The terms *salt* and *sodium* are often used interchangeably, but, in fact, salt (also known as *sodium chloride*) contains both sodium and chloride.

Salt can easily be controlled in the foods we eat. Review these tips on reducing your overall intake:

- Limit table salt added to foods during preparation.
- Remove the saltshaker from the table. When you shake you have no idea how much is coming out.
- Select canned vegetables, soups, and broths without added salt.
- Limit intake of processed foods and luncheon meats.
- Keep your eye open for nutrition labels on processed dinners, convenience foods, crackers, chips, nuts and seeds, all known to contribute extra sodium.
- Watch your condiments—ketchup, barbecue sauce, soy sauce, pickles and relish, olives, mustard—all guilty of containing sodium.
- Substitute herbs and spices for salt in flavoring foods.

## If You Drink Alcohol, Do So in Moderation

The final dietary guideline offers a message about alcohol consumption. Although not considered a food, alcoholic beverages do contain calories but no other nutrients.

When consumed in large amounts, drinking alcohol can be harmful, even dangerous. A high consumption of alcohol can lead to various health problems including high blood pressure, heart disease, stomach and liver problems, and brain damage. And because of its high caloric content, drinking excessive alcoholic beverages can contribute to problems with obesity. Other risks of alcohol consumption result in impaired judgment and decreased motor responses that can lead to serious accidents when driving.

Some research does indicate health benefits of moderate consumption of certain types of alcoholic beverages. Studies have shown a decrease in heart disease as a result. But this is not a reason to begin drinking. Recommendations continue to suggest limiting consumption to no more than one drink each day for women and two drinks each day for men.

An alcoholic drink refers to any of the following:

- 1 ounce (80 proof) distilled spirits (70 calories)
- 12 ounces regular beer (150 calories)
- 12 ounces light beer (90 calories)
- 4 ounces wine (80 calories)
- 2 ounces sherry (75 calories)

Eating healthfully is all about choosing foods wisely and making good choices. Learning about the various options you have in selecting your diet helps you make the best choices for your particular needs. Understanding the messages brought forth in the Dietary Guidelines for Americans can help in doing just that. As we continue, more information about your particular food choices will be shared. You will learn to choose healthy foods, and by doing so, you will greatly increase your chances of living a healthier and active life. If you do not, other consequences may arise. The choice is yours.

## CHAPTER 6
# *Smart Eating/ Smart Snacking*

Choosing to eat smart sets the stage for the healthiest way you can lose weight over the long run. It involves no deprivation, no restrictions, just choosing a wide variety of foods throughout three meals and one to two snacks each day.

# The Food Guide Pyramid

Learning about nutrition is simpler today than ever before. Back in the early 1990s, the United States Department of Agriculture (USDA), in cooperation with the Department of Health and Human Services, created a visual tool for teaching people about good nutrition. This tool is called the Food Guide Pyramid. It is used to help people of all ages plan and create healthy diets according to guidelines established from the Recommended Dietary Allowances and the Dietary Guidelines for Americans.

**FIGURE 5-1:**
The USDA Food Guide Pyramid

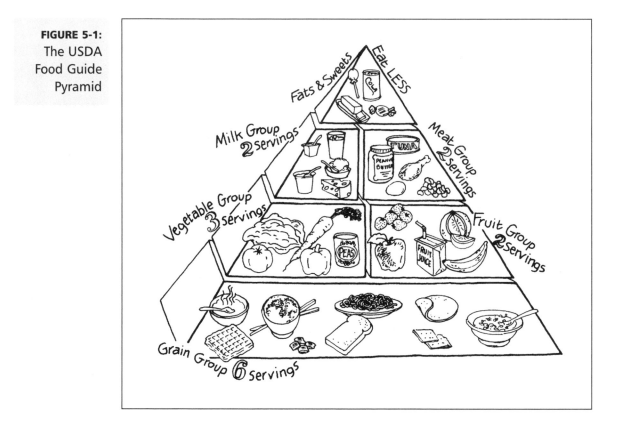

The Food Guide Pyramid divides food into five main food groups (starches, fruits, vegetables, dairy, and meats). A recommended number of servings from each group and appropriate portion sizes are provided to help people balance their food intake, choose a variety of foods, and consume all foods in moderation.

Balancing food choices means selecting foods from each of the different groups for various meals and snacks each day. Some foods may be higher in fat, sodium, sugars or calories, whereas others will be lower. For example, a balanced meal could include a hamburger patty on a bun with lettuce, tomato, and pickles, a tossed salad, and strawberry slices. Here you have balanced the "higher fat" hamburger patty from the meat group with the lower-fat vegetable and fruit choices.

Selecting a variety of foods means you should select different options from each of the food groups during the day in order to obtain a wide range of the different nutrients that can be found in each group. For example, all vegetables are great choices, but dark green vegetables provide different types of vitamins than orange ones. Choosing an orange food like baby carrot sticks at lunch and a green food like broccoli at dinner will ensure that you obtain the various types of vitamins.

Moderation means that you should watch your portion sizes. Any and all foods are allowed, but eating too much of a food is not a good idea. Even the healthiest of food choices, like milk, for example, can be unhealthy if consumed in too-large portions.

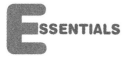

**ESSENTIALS** Different foods supply different nutrients. No single food can supply every nutrient your body needs. This is why we need to eat a variety of foods each day.

## The Bread/Starch Group

The Food Guide Pyramid is built on the premise that the bottom is larger in order to illustrate that we should eat more from this group than the others. The bread, cereal, rice, and pasta group (often called the grain, or starch, group) forms the basis of a healthy diet.

The range of servings from this group each day should be between six to eleven servings. Teenagers and more highly active adults may need nine to eleven servings due to their growth and activity needs; elderly and sedentary individuals may require only six servings each day. Foods from this group provide an excellent source of energy and offer many complex carbohydrates and fiber, and thus they should provide over 50 percent of a person's daily energy and caloric needs.

## The Vegetable and Fruit Groups

The vegetable and fruit groups are evenly distributed as you move up the pyramid. Here, you will find a large number of food choices that provide important sources of vitamins, minerals, and fiber. Three to four servings should be eaten daily from the vegetable group and two to four selections from the fruit group.

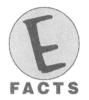

**FACTS**

In the Food Guide Pyramid, the grain group, vegetable group, and fruit group provide almost three-quarters of recommended daily consumption.

## The Protein Groups (Dairy and Meats)

Dairy foods and the sources of meat products both are high in protein. These are also lined up together on the next tier of the pyramid. Dairy food choices supply protein as well as calcium and other important vitamins and minerals, including milk, cheese, yogurt, and cottage cheese. The meat group, also high in protein, iron, and other minerals, includes foods like beef, poultry, fish, dried beans and peas, nuts, and eggs. Recommended servings from the dairy group are two to three servings daily, while a total of 5 and 7 ounces are suggested from the meat group.

## Fats and Sugars

The very top of the pyramid is reserved for the extra foods that do not fit into any other food group. These include fats, sugars, oils, and sweets, such as candy, soft drinks, butter, margarine, cakes, cookies, and many convenience-type snack foods. These foods provide very little, if any, nutritional value and consumption should be limited. Often these foods are referred to as those "empty calorie" foods because they provide us with calories but few, if any, other nutrients.

Overall dietary recommendations established with the Food Guide Pyramid promotes a healthy diet, high in carbohydrates (particularly complex ones), and low in sugars and fats. Further information shared here will offer you insight on using the pyramid to the best of your abilities as an aide to maintaining your health and body weight.

# Daily Serving Recommendations

Certain daily recommendations are provided for each food group in the form of a range. The exact number of servings that you will need from each of these groups depends on many factors, including your age, size, gender, health status, and activity level. Young children and teenagers often require additional foods because of their body's needs during the growing years. Athletes may require more servings due to their high energy needs. Sedentary individuals and the elderly often require less because of their less-active lifestyle. And individuals seeking to lose weight may reduce their recommended serving suggestions in order to decrease overall consumption.

Here is a breakdown of recommended daily servings for maintaining health:

| FOOD GROUP | CALORIE LEVEL* | | |
| --- | --- | --- | --- |
| | 1,600 CALORIES | 2,200 CALORIES | 2,800 CALORIES |
| Grain/Starch Group | 6 servings | 9 servings | 11 servings |
| Vegetable Group | 3 servings | 4 servings | 5 servings |
| Fruit Group | 2 servings | 3 servings | 4 servings |
| Dairy Group** | 2–3 servings | 2–3 servings | 2–3 servings |
| Meat/Protein Group | 5 ounces | 6 ounces | 7 ounces |
| Fats/Oils/Sweets Group | use sparingly | use sparingly | use sparingly |

*1,600 calories is adequate for most sedentary women and some elderly adults
2,200 calories is adequate for most children, teenage girls, lightly active women, and sedentary men.
2,800 calories is adequate for teenage boys, many active men, and some very active women.
**Teenagers would require additional servings from the dairy group to help support growth and development.

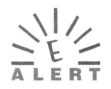

## Daily Serving Recommendations for Weight Reduction

Now, let's see how we can modify the recommended daily servings for losing weight. The most effective way to lose weight is to do so with gradual decreases in calorie requirements. This will allow for a slow and steady weight loss. Caloric decreases should be no more than 500–700 calories per day. At this level, individuals can expect a weight loss of about 1 to 2 pounds per week.

| FOOD GROUP | CALORIE LEVEL* | | |
| --- | --- | --- | --- |
| | 1,200 CALORIES | 1,500 CALORIES | 1,800 CALORIES |
| Grain/Starch Group | 5 servings | 6 servings | 8 servings |
| Vegetable Group | 3 servings | 4 servings | 5 servings |
| Fruit Group | 2 servings | 3 servings | 4 servings |
| Dairy Group | 2 servings | 2 servings | 2 servings |
| Meat/Protein Group | 5 ounces | 6 ounces | 7 ounces |
| Fats/Oils/Sweets Group | limit to 1/day | limit to 1–2/day | limit to 2/day |

By decreasing one or two servings from each group, you are continuing to offer yourself the benefits of a healthy, well-rounded diet. Your body will continue to receive the many nutrients it needs, but it will also receive less overall calories. This will contribute to a slow, but permanent, weight loss.

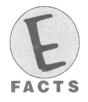

To effectively lose weight, calorie decreases should not exceed 500 to 700 calories per day. This daily reduction should bring on a weight loss of approximately 1 to 2 pounds per week.

# How Much Is a Serving?

Just knowing how many servings we should eat from each food group is not enough. We also need to know how large each of these servings should be. This is a big effort for many people. We are all guilty of saying "I really don't eat that much," when in reality we may have eaten two, three, or even four portions at one sitting. Understanding the proper serving size can be tricky. However, it also is one of the most important details you can learn when trying to control your food intake and help lose those extra pounds.

A serving size is defined as the amount of food that should be eaten at one time. These serving sizes can, and do, add up quickly. People may think that six to eleven servings from the grain group sounds like a lot of food, but they may easily be consuming twice that amount without even realizing it. Visualizing a serving is often difficult. Measuring one is a better option, at least until you understand and can better calculate an appropriate serving size. This will help you to more accurately estimate servings eaten in the course of a day.

**E**SSENTIALS    Initially a food scale and set of measuring cups and spoons will help determine accurate serving sizes. After a while, estimating portions will become second nature.

In the **BREAD/STARCH GROUP**, any of the following is considered one serving:

- 1 slice bread
- ½ hamburger/hot dog bun
- ½ small bagel or English muffin
- 1 small dinner roll, biscuit or muffin
- 5 small crackers
- 2 graham crackers
- ¾ to 1 cup (about 1 ounce) ready-to-eat cereal
- ½ cup cooked cereal, rice or pasta

- 1 (4-inch) pita bread
- 1 (8-inch) flour or corn tortilla
- 2 corn taco shells
- 3 hard breadsticks (about 4 inches long)
- 1 soft breadstick (about 6 inches long)
- 2 long pretzel rods or 8 three-ring pretzels
- 1 large or 5 mini-rice cakes
- 2 cups air-popped popcorn
- 12 baked chips

In the **VEGETABLE GROUP**, one serving is any of the following:

- ½ cup chopped raw or cooked vegetables
- 1 cup leafy raw vegetable
- 1 medium tomato or 6 cherry tomatoes
- 8 baby carrot sticks or 1 large carrot stick
- ½ medium cucumber
- 1 medium ear corn-on-the-cob
- 1 medium baked potato
- 1 small or ½ large sweet potato
- 10 snow peas
- 2 broccoli spears
- 6 asparagus spears
- 1 medium pepper (green, red, yellow)
- 1 artichoke
- 4 Brussels sprouts
- ¾ cup vegetable juice
- ½ cup tomato or pasta sauce
- ½ cup tomato paste
- 1 cup vegetable soup

In the **FRUIT GROUP**, one serving is any of the following:

- 1 medium apple, banana, orange, peach, pear, nectarine, or similar fruit

- ½ grapefruit
- ¼ melon wedge (¼ cantaloupe or ⅛ honeydew)
- 6 strawberries
- 10 Bing cherries
- 12 grapes
- 2 clementines or apricots
- ½ mango
- ¼ papaya
- 1 kiwi
- ½ cup canned fruit
- ½ cup cut-up fresh fruit
- ½ cup frozen fruit
- ¼ cup dried fruit
- ¾ cup fruit juice

In the **DAIRY GROUP**, one serving is any of the following:

- 1 cup milk or buttermilk
- 8 ounces yogurt
- 1½ ounces natural cheese
- 2 ounces processed cheese
- 1 cup cottage cheese
- ½ cup ricotta cheese
- ½ cup nonfat dry milk powder
- ½ cup evaporated (skim) milk
- 1 cup frozen yogurt
- 1½ cups ice milk

In the **MEAT GROUP**, one serving is any of the following:

- 2½ to 3 ounces cooked lean meat, poultry, pork, veal, or fish
- 2 to 3 ounces canned fish, tuna, or salmon

The following count as a third of a meat serving or the equivalent to 1 ounce:

- ½ cup cooked beans
- 2 tablespoons peanut butter
- ½ cup tofu
- 1 egg
- ¼ cup sunflower seeds, pumpkin seeks
- ¼ cup chopped nuts, walnuts, pecans, peanuts
- ½ cup baked beans
- 1 ounce Canadian bacon or lean ham
- 1 hot dog
- 6 medium shrimp
- ⅓ cup canned crabmeat or clams
- ½ cup canned lobster or shrimp

In the **FATS/OILS/SWEETS GROUP**, these are each one serving:

- 1 teaspoon margarine, butter, oil, mayonnaise
- 2 teaspoons diet margarine or reduced-fat mayonnaise
- 1 tablespoon salad dressing
- 2 tablespoons reduced-fat salad dressing
- 1 tablespoon cream cheese
- 1 tablespoon sour cream
- 2 tablespoons whipped topping

The following are **FREE FOODS** (they do not fall into any specific group and offer less than 20 calories/serving):

- broth/bouillon
- ketchup (1 tablespoon)
- coffee/tea/iced tea
- diet, calorie-free soft drinks and beverages
- diet syrup
- hot sauces
- lemon

- lime
- low-sugar jams/jellies (2 teaspoons)
- mustard
- nonstick pan sprays
- soy sauce
- spices/herbs
- sugar-free hard candies/gum
- sugar substitutes
- unsweetened gelatin
- unsweetened pickles
- vinegar
- Worcestershire sauce
- celery
- cucumbers
- green onions
- lettuce (iceberg/romaine/spinach)
- mushrooms
- radishes

Initially, it is important to measure rather than to just "eyeball" servings to be the most accurate with your measurements. After a while you will find it much easier to estimate serving sizes. Some people find it helpful to visualize a common household item for proper measurement.

| ONE SERVING OF . . . | IS ABOUT THE SIZE OF . . . |
| --- | --- |
| Pasta/rice | an ice cream scoop |
| Hamburger patty | a deck of cards |
| Chicken breast | a fisted hand |
| Cooked vegetable/canned fruit | a small custard cup |
| Fresh fruit | a tennis ball |
| Cheese | a computer diskette or the size of a thumb |
| Butter/margarine/cream cheese | tip of a thumb |
| Snack foods | no more than a handful |

## It All Takes Planning

Try to begin to plan your meals and your snacks by using what you have learned so far with the Food Guide Pyramid. Meal planning with the Food Guide Pyramid helps you make wise food choices while doing so in adequate portions.

### Logging Food Intake

First begin by logging everything you eat within a three-day period. You can create your own chart, or you can use the charts found in Chapter 3 or at the end of this book. This log is your diet diary. By keeping track of your intake, you can determine if you are getting an appropriate amount of calories and the various other nutrients you need on a daily basis. (It is always best to jot down your intake immediately after you have eaten it, otherwise it may be difficult to remember everything you have consumed, including condiments, beverages, and snacks. And don't forget to include bites taken over the stove when cooking or when cleaning up the dishes.) You can then compare your intake to the Food Guide Pyramid to determine whether you are consuming the appropriate number of servings from each group. Along with jotting down the foods you eat, you can also fill in a chart determining how many servings from each group you need each day. This helps you determine your needs and requirements at a glance and offers you insight into what additional foods you need to eat during the course of a day's time.

FIGURE 6-2 shows a sample plan for a 1,500-calorie intake.

During the day, as you consume a particular food, check off the group in which it can be found. For example, if you had half of a bagel, a banana, and a glass of milk for breakfast, you would mark off a box in the grain, fruit, and dairy groups. Then for lunch, if you eat a turkey sandwich, carrot sticks and half of a cantaloupe, you would mark off a meat, two breads, a vegetable, and a fruit. Make sure you see which groups you are eating too many foods from and those you are not eating enough from so you can better plan your meals and snacks.

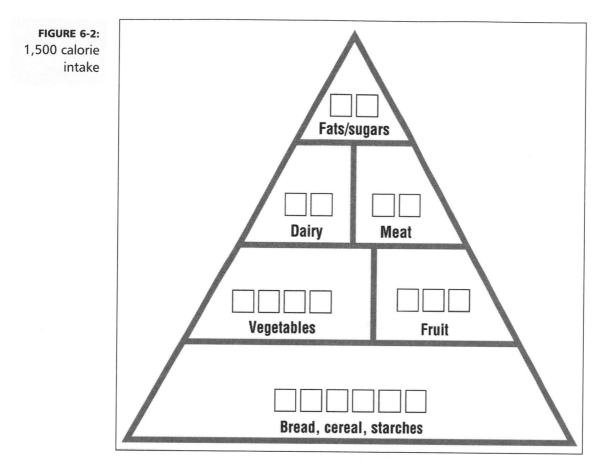

**FIGURE 6-2:**
1,500 calorie intake

So now as you plan for dinner and additional snacks, keep in mind that you need some meat or protein and some additional vegetables. Your fruit allotment for the day is almost complete, so remember this as you continue eating for the remainder of the day. Also keep in mind that any fat or oil used in food preparation or added to food, like margarine in pasta, needs to be recorded as well. Refer to this chart often to help you determine your food group needs. I have incorporated this check-off list into the diet diary at the end of the book to help you on a day-to-day basis.

If you also find that you are frequently eating out of boredom, loneliness, or stress, you can jot down your moods as well. This will help you keep track of your responses to various moods. For example, whenever you have an argument with your spouse, you may find your hand in the cookie jar. This is a reaction to a behavior that you may need to better control. Also, if you find that in the late evening you are bored with the programs on television or don't have a hobby or book to read, and a dish of ice cream begins to fill the void, then you may want to schedule some evening activities with friends or plan to walk the dog during this time.

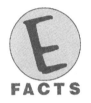

**FACTS**

A food diary is a tool or record that keeps track of the kinds and amounts of foods and beverages you consume on a daily or weekly basis. Diet professionals can track caloric and nutrient levels through these diaries as well as observe problems associated with eating patterns.

## Your Best Food Options

I can also offer you many helpful suggestions on selecting foods from the various food groups that will give you healthier and wiser choices. Lean meats, poultry without skin, and reduced-fat products are just some of the wiser selections.

In the Bread/Starch Group, aim for whole grain/bran breads/muffins/bagels/cereals, higher fiber ready-to-eat cereals with low sugar content, and brown rice. In the Vegetable Group, try to incorporate lots of fresh vegetables (which provide greater amounts of fiber) and plain frozen vegetables (limit those with sauces). In the Fruit Group, eat lots of fresh fruits (with skin). They provide greater fiber benefits than canned fruits or juices. If you choose canned fruits, they should be packed in water or fruit juice without added sugar. In the Dairy Group, look for low-fat and fat-free dairy products, including milk, yogurt, cottage, and ricotta cheese; reduced-fat cheeses (as a substitute for regular sliced and shredded cheese); plain yogurt as a substitute for sour cream; and low-fat frozen yogurt and ice milk (as a good alternative to ice cream). In the Meat Group, choose lean cuts of meat with little visible fat or marbling; white meat chicken and poultry (which contain less fat than dark meat); skinless poultry or poultry with the skin removed before eating; lower-fat processed luncheon meats like bologna, salami, hot dogs; and canned fish packed in water, not vegetable oil. And in the Fats/Oils/Sweets Group, you should aim for moderate-sized portions of lower-fat margarine spreads; lower-fat salad dressings and mayonnaise; low-calorie soft drinks; and lower-fat cookies and pastries. (Be cautious of these products, though, because many of them are not really lower in overall calories.)

**E**SSENTIALS    When selecting foods at all calorie levels, choose lean and lower-fat foods in all food groups, limit the consumption of extra fat, and reduce the consumption of "empty calorie" foods.

## Healthy Snack Choices

It's not only necessary to choose meals that fit into the overall food pyramid. Snacks should be chosen from the food groups as well. Snacking refers to the consumption of foods that occurs between the three main meals each day. Most people eat at least one snack daily, and many people snack constantly throughout the course of a day. The snack-food industry is a fast-growing market, and many foods are added to selections available each year. Food manufacturers know that adults and children alike are intrigued by the snacks sold at the grocery stores and that people often buy many of these convenience-type foods to keep handy at home.

But it is not so difficult to alter your eating and buying habits to incorporate healthy snacks. The most important thing to remember is to eat snacks that are nutrient-dense rather than those that are "empty-calorie" choices. Nutrient-dense foods are ones that offer quality nutrition, vitamins, minerals, fiber, protein, or other nutrients in addition to calories. Again, those empty-calorie foods offer calories but no other nutrition. Foods selected for snacks should be ones that come out of the various groups in the Food Guide Pyramid, not just the Fats/Oils/Sweet Group.

Keep this in mind next time you grab for that cookie or candy bar. Wouldn't a piece of fruit or some yogurt be a better choice?

Healthy snack options include the following:

- Fresh/dried fruit
- Fresh vegetable sticks
- Cheese cubes/cheese stick
- Air-popped popcorn
- Pretzels
- Bagel/pita chips
- Mini-muffins
- Raisin bread

- Fruit-filled bars
- Graham crackers
- Rice cakes
- Baked chips
- Peanut butter on crackers or celery
- Low-fat yogurt
- Frozen yogurt/ice milk
- Cottage cheese

Planning your meals and snacks is an essential step in beginning a lifelong plan of healthy eating and ultimately in your controlling body weight. The Food Guide Pyramid is just one tool that can be helpful to you when planning for the dietary needs of yourself and your family. Not only does this tool assist in creating a healthy diet, it offers guidance on balance, variety, and moderation as well. This tool is also helpful in creating the basis for reducing food intake for overall weight control. As you continue to learn more about nutrition, you will find additional ways to put more of this information into practice.

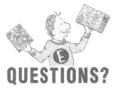

**QUESTIONS?**

**What is a nutrient-dense food?**
Nutrient-dense foods are those that contribute nutrients like vitamins, minerals, and fiber as well as calories. These foods can be found within the grain, vegetable, fruit, dairy, and meat groups of the Food Guide Pyramid.

CHAPTER 7

# What's the Best Way to Lose?

Obesity affects one in every three Americans, and as a result over half of the American population seek results through some type of diet or weight-loss program each year. Few of these people really understand how and what they should be doing.

## Are You Ready to Lose?

So are you ready to lose those excess pounds for good? Have you decided it's now time to focus on health and good nutrition and a slow but steady weight loss? If so, ask yourself the following questions:

- Am I ready to make changes to my lifestyle?
- Am I willing to take my time losing weight?
- Do I understand my eating patterns need to be permanent, not temporary?
- Do I understand that the weight will come off slowly?
- Am I willing to increase my activity level?
- Am I willing to plan my meals and snacks?
- Am I motivated to start this time?

**ALERT**

Remember: You should not be following a "diet." You should be aiming toward eating healthy!

If you answered yes to all of these questions, you're ready to begin. Take it slow. Do it right.

## Losing Weight Safely and Effectively

Losing weight safely and effectively requires an approach that includes setting goals (both short-term and long-term goals), changing eating habits, and incorporating physical activity into daily life.

### Set Those Goals

Your first step should be to set some goals. Make them realistic—ones you know you can strive to meet, but ones that will challenge you along the way. You should be losing weight for yourself and not for anyone else—not for your spouse, your mother, or your best friend. You must have a positive attitude, too. Remember that short-term goals set your plans for the upcoming week or month—they are attainable. Long-term goals should not be impossible, but they should challenge and motivate you to keep striving for success. These are goals that you may want to accomplish in six months or a year. If you didn't get a chance to make some goals earlier, do so now. Ask yourself:

- What do I want to accomplish is the next week?
- What do I want to accomplish in the next month?
- What do I want to accomplish in the next year?

**ESSENTIALS**

Be realistic with your goals. If they are too hard to accomplish, you may get frustrated and never meet them.

## Lose Slowly

Initially your weight-loss goal should be to lose weight slowly. Make small changes. Don't expect drastic results at first. To lose weight slowly, plan to lose no more than 1 to 2 pounds each week. This can be accomplished by reducing caloric intake by about 500 calories each day.

Here's how. One pound is the equivalence of 3,500 calories. To gain a pound, you will need to eat an additional 3,500 calories. To lose a pound, you need to eat a deficit of 3,500 calories. An average person who consumes 2,000 calories per day to maintain his weight would have to increase his caloric intake to 2,500 each day (an additional 500 calories) over a week's time to gain a pound. On the contrary, the opposite is true to lose. This person would have to decrease his caloric intake to 1,500 calories each day (minus 500 calories) over a week's time to lose a pound.

Physical activity can also be counted into the equation. (For more information on exercise, see Chapter 19.) The more you move, the more you burn off.

The first adjustments to your overall diet will also bring on some fluid loss. This may add an extra weight loss of 1 to 2 pounds the first week (as fluids), but this will be only temporary. If weight loss efforts are continued, about 1 to 2 pounds can be lost per week. This is a healthy and adequate weight loss for any person.

So wouldn't it be great if you lost 1 pound per week for three months? That's about 12 pounds. In six months, that would make about 25 pounds, and in one year, that totals 50 pounds. Think about the last year and reflect on all the so-called diets you have tried. Isn't it now worth the time to do it right and get it off once and for all?

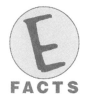

**FACTS**

A weight loss of 1 to 2 pounds per week is usually safe and considered adequate. To lose weight most effectively, a modest reduction of 500 calories per day is suggested to result in an average loss of 1 pound per week.

## Examining Your Attitude about Food

In order to be successful in your attempts to lose weight and keep it off permanently, you need to have a good attitude about food. Here you can find direction on working on your new approach.

Make health your first priority. Whenever you waver about your dietary changes, think about how much you are doing for your health.

Think in terms of "healthy eating," not dieting. Restrictive dieting is a temporary state. Healthy eating is a lifelong approach. Learn to make permanent changes.

Set your direction. The more direction you set for yourself, the more you will aim to accomplish.

Be sure to write down your goals. Post them, and check up on yourself regularly. Having your goals with scheduled dates posted on the refrigerator becomes a constant reminder and one that you will see every time you reach to open the door. Post these in other places too, if it helps.

Keep positive. You're doing this for yourself, not someone else. Keep upbeat and focused. Accept praise for your successes and accomplishments. Feel good about yourself, and people around you will notice. Remember you're not perfect. Slip-ups will occur. Just don't let them get you down. Get over it and start again.

Make your eating approach one that works for you and your lifestyle. Plan meals and snacks to fit into your busy day's schedule. If you have an early appointment at work and do not have time for breakfast, pack a high-energy snack (like a mini-bagel and orange juice box) for the commute to work. If you go to the park with your kids, pack some snacks like raisins, an apple, or some pretzels. These snacks will help curb your appetite and keep you from being drawn to the ice-cream man or other convenience-type snacks. And don't sacrifice eating altogether. You will only set yourself up for failure later.

Keep in mind that there are no "good foods" and no "bad foods," only good and bad eating plans. If you want to splurge sometime, do so. Just make sure you plan for it. One splurge doesn't need to feed another. Everyone is entitled to a treat. Just compensate by eating lower-fat foods during the days when you know you will be eating higher-fat foods in the evening.

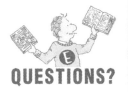

**QUESTIONS?**

**Is it okay to eat after dinner?**
Yes, but use your common sense on what and how much you consume based on your daily allotment. Keep in mind that large amounts of food late at night or foods high in fat and calories aren't a wise choice, particularly when you are less active. Consider higher-fiber fruits and vegetables, fruit smoothies, or graham crackers and milk as an option.

## Seeking a Plan That Works for You

You may think the Food Guide Pyramid focuses solely on healthy eating, not weight loss, but in fact it does both. Your main objective in reducing your food intake is to do so while choosing foods from all the food groups.

Don't forget the importance of balance, variety, and moderation, too. Those words should help to start making necessary dietary changes. Remember, balance means selecting foods from each of the different food groups for your meals and snacks each day. Selecting a variety of foods means choosing different options from each of the food groups in order to obtain a variety of nutrients each day. And moderation means keeping portion sizes adequate. And as you select foods, keep them lower in fat and higher in fiber.

| FOOD GROUP | 1,200 CALORIES | 1,500 CALORIES | 1,800 CALORIES |
| --- | --- | --- | --- |
| Grain/Starch Group | 5 servings | 6 servings | 8 servings |
| Vegetable Group | 3 servings | 4 servings | 5 servings |
| Fruit Group | 2 servings | 3 servings | 4 servings |
| Dairy Group | 2 servings | 2 servings | 2 servings |
| Meat/Protein Group | 5 ounces | 6 ounces | 7 ounces |
| Fat/Oils/Sweets Group | limit to 1/day | limit to 1–2/day | limit to 2/day |

Although it is not really necessary to count calories, it is important to understand the calorie contributions of various foods. Be careful not to cut your intake too low. It is not safe to decrease your intake to fewer than 1,200 calories. In the meantime, strive for a plan that works for you.

Be smart with weight loss. Any plan you choose should do all the following:

- Be safe. It should offer sufficient calories and include the recommended dietary allowances for vitamins, minerals, and protein.
- Offer a slow and steady weight loss. Loss of ½ to 2 pounds per week is adequate.
- Alter lifestyle habits. Changes to eating and exercise patterns are essential in order to eliminate problems that may have contributed to weight gain.
- Include direction for weight maintenance after initial weight goal is achieved. There is no benefit to losing the weight if you regain it. Weight maintenance can be as difficult as weight loss.
- Seek support assistance and keep educated. Learning along the way is key to living a healthier and happier life.

Let's focus in on a specific plan. Here you can divide the recommendations from the above chart into your meals and snacks each day.

| FOOD GROUP | 1,200 CALORIES | 1,500 CALORIES | 1,800 CALORIES |
|---|---|---|---|
| **BREAKFAST** | | | |
| Grain/Starch | 1 serving | 1 serving | 2 servings |
| Fruit | 1 serving | 1 serving | 1 serving |
| Dairy | 1 serving | 1 serving | 1 serving |
| Protein | 0 | 0 | 1 ounce |
| **SNACK** | | | |
| Fruit | — | — | 1 serving |
| **LUNCH** | | | |
| Grain/Starch | 2 servings | 2 servings | 2 servings |
| Vegetable | 1 serving | 2 servings | 2 servings |
| Fruit | — | 1 serving | 1 serving |
| Protein | 2 ounces | 3 ounces | 3 ounces |
| Fat | — | — | 1 serving |
| **SNACK** | | | |
| Starch | 1 serving | 1 serving | 1 serving |
| **DINNER** | | | |
| Grain/Starch | 1 serving | 2 servings | 2 servings |
| Vegetable | 2 servings | 2 servings | 2 servings |
| Fruit | — | — | 1 serving |
| Protein | 3 ounces | 3 ounces | 3 ounces |
| Fat | 1 serving | 1 serving | 1 serving |
| **SNACK** | | | |
| Starch | — | — | 1 serving |
| Fruit | 1 serving | 1 serving | 1 serving |
| Dairy | 1 serving | 1 serving | 1 serving |

Now here's how you can incorporate foods into the plan. Here you can find an outline of food selections for each plan.

| FOOD GROUP | 1,200 CALORIES | 1,500 CALORIES | 1,800 CALORIES |
|---|---|---|---|
| **BREAKFAST** | | | |
| Grain/Starch | 1 oz. dry cereal | 1 oz. dry cereal | 2 slices toast + jam |
| Fruit | ¾ c. orange juice | ¾ c. orange juice | ¾ c. orange juice |
| Dairy | 1 c. low-fat milk | 1 c. low-fat milk | 1 cup low-fat milk |
| Protein | — | — | 1 scrambled egg |
| **SNACK** | | | |
| Grain/Starch | — | — | small banana |
| **LUNCH** | | | |
| Grain/Starch | 2 slices bread | 2 slices bread | 2 slices bread |
| Vegetable | sliced tomato/lettuce | sliced tomato/lettuce | sliced tomato/lettuce |
| | — | ½ c. coleslaw | ½ c. coleslaw |
| Fruit | — | ¼ cantaloupe wedge | ¼ cantaloupe wedge |
| Protein | 2 oz. sliced turkey | 3 oz. sliced turkey | 3 oz. sliced turkey |
| Fat | — | — | 1 tsp. mayonnaise |
| **SNACK** | | | |
| Grain/Starch | 2 graham crackers | 2 graham crackers | 2 graham crackers |
| **DINNER** | | | |
| Grain/Starch | ½ c. rice | ½ c. rice | ½ c. rice |
| | — | dinner roll | dinner roll |
| Vegetable | broccoli spears | broccoli spears | broccoli spears |
| | garden salad | garden salad | garden salad |
| Fruit | — | — | ½ c. strawberries |
| Protein | 3 oz. salmon fillet | 3 oz. salmon fillet | 3 oz. salmon fillet |
| Fat | 2 Tbsp. reduced-fat salad dressing | 2 Tbsp. reduced-fat salad dressing | 2 Tbsp. reduced-fat salad dressing |
| **SNACK** | | | |
| Grain/Starch | — | — | 2 c. popcorn |
| Fruit | smoothie made with: 1 c. low-fat milk + ½ c. frozen blueberries | smoothie made with: 1 c. low-fat milk + ½ c. frozen blueberries | smoothie made with: 1 c. low-fat milk + ½ c. frozen blueberries |

If you find the 1,200-caloric plan too restrictive, add an additional fruit or some vegetables. Or work between two different plans throughout the week depending on your hunger and schedule.

There are also many free-type foods that do not fit into any of the groups, as they are considered bonus choices. These foods do not have significant calories or nutrition, but they are good for helping to fill you up and satisfying hunger pangs. Add these selections throughout your day as necessary. Some food choices you may enjoy are dill pickles, sliced cucumbers, fresh green beans, unsweetened gelatin, calorie-free soft drinks and beverages, sugar-free hard candies or gum, and broth or bouillon. For a more extensive listing of the "free" foods, refer to the list in Chapter 6.

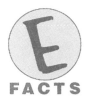

**FACTS**

Foods are definitely metabolized differently at different times of the day. Foods consumed at breakfast are quickly metabolized (burned) because physical activity usually follows this meal. Large meals eaten late at night are not metabolized as well because resting at night requires little activity.

More calorie plans offering meal and snack suggestions can be found in Chapter 18.

## Setting Some Weight-Loss Rules

Each and every person will find different ways to control their food intake. It helps to create a set of rules to live by. In this section, I give you some that you can incorporate into your plan to help you on the road to reduction.

Plan your meals and snacks. Write all foods down ahead of time if you need to. Then you will know what to buy and what to prepare.

Don't skip meals. Eat at regular times each day. Eating haphazardly leads to impulse snacking and increased opportunities for failure.

Sit down when you eat. Pick a spot, most likely at the kitchen table, where all your meals and snacks will be eaten. When you grab an impulsive snack, you may then ask yourself, is it worth it to sit down and enjoy this now?

Avoid outside distractions. Turn off the television, push the newspaper aside, and hang up the telephone. Any outside disturbance will cause you to consume more than you realize.

Measure and portion out your foods at the stove and carry them over to the table. This will help control second portions—and who needs two meals at one sitting, anyway? To be sure you don't go back for more, wrap up the leftovers before you begin to eat.

Take your time eating. Enjoy the good taste of food. It takes about twenty minutes from the time you begin eating until the time your stomach can signal your brain that you are full. By eating slowly, you will often consume less, because you begin to feel fuller.

Don't worry about cleaning your plate. We no longer expect you to be a member of the "clean your plate club." If you are full, stop eating. Save the rest of your food for later, if you like.

Try filling up on a cup of broth or some raw vegetables to curb an excessive appetite at the beginning of a meal. These "free" foods are filling.

Keep your diary. When you jot down the foods you eat, you tend to eat less overall. Keeping track of your intake is a sure way you will be aware of what you are eating. It also can help professionals, like registered dietitians, evaluate your downfalls and problems you may encounter along the way.

**E**SSENTIALS

Don't forget snacks when reducing food intake. Find snacks that fit into your overall eating plan. Low-fat choices like bagel chips, pretzels, graham crackers, fresh fruits, raisins, and raw vegetables.

## Seeing How Small Changes Add Up

There are so many ways to cut excess calories from your daily intake that you may be surprised how easy it can really be. At first cutting back 500 calories or so each day may seem extreme, but 50 or 100 calories at a time might be a cut you can easily accomplish. (That's just one cookie or the savings from substituting skim for whole milk.) Here are some other smart alternatives:

- Eat an open-faced sandwich (1 slice of bread, for savings of 70 calories)
- Drink black coffee (1 tsp. sugar and 1 Tbsp. cream, for savings of 36 calories)
- Choose steamed white or brown rice over fried rice (savings of 100 calories)
- Substitute light mayonnaise over regular, or better yet no mayonnaise (savings of 65–100 calories)
- Crunch on ten carrot sticks instead of ten potato chips (savings of 70 calories)
- Drink skim milk over 2 percent or whole (savings of 20–50 calories)
- Try plain low-fat yogurt with added fresh fruit in place of fruited yogurt (savings of 50 calories)
- Make a banana smoothie instead of a milkshake (savings of 50 calories)
- Snack on a vanilla wafer over a chocolate chip cookie (savings of 75 calories)
- Treat yourself with angel food cake, not devil's food cake (savings of 200 calories)

# Looking at Commercial Weight-Loss Programs

Some people like to plan their programs themselves. Many others feel the need to get some outside help and support when it comes to losing weight. This is a personal and individual decision for each and everyone.

## What Can a Program Offer?

Consumers interested in seeking out additional support through an established weight-loss program should select a program that offers behavior modification and psychological support. The program should focus its efforts on long-term weight loss and management, helpful instruction including nutrition guidance and meal planning, recommendation for increased activity, and motivational assistance. It should also demonstrate evidence of past success both initially and over the long term.

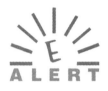

Be cautious of so-called nutrition experts. When seeking outside help, look for a registered dietitian who has a background in foods and nutrition and possibly a specialty in weight control.

Some programs require weekly visits, and some have less frequent requirements. Some programs require the purchase of special foods and gadgets, and others do not. Still others may put you under strict physician supervision, while others may not. Before you make the decision to begin a specific program, consider the following checklist.

## A Checklist for Choosing an Adequate Weight-Loss Program

If you choose to seek out a commercial weight-loss program, ask yourself the following questions. Does it:

- Offer a variety of food choices from all food groups?
- Include foods you enjoy as well as those easily available in the grocery store?
- Recommend changes that fit into your lifestyle?
- Is the plan affordable—worth it to you financially?
- Offer recommendations for increasing physical activity?
- Motivate you—build up your self-esteem?

If you determine that the answer is "yes" to all of the above questions, you are on your way toward choosing an adequate weight-loss program.

## The Best Program for You

After you consider your options with a commercial weight-loss program, find the one that works best for you. Make an appointment to talk to a representative from that program. Also, try to talk to other individuals who have joined. Ask about the following:

- What are the success and failure rates?
- What makes this program better than others?
- Who instructs participants on diet and nutrition? Is this person trained, a professional or not?
- How often are visits required?
- Are there any health risks for going on this program?
- Do you have to buy special foods, meals, dietary supplements, or gadgets?
- Can you buy regular foods at the supermarket?
- Can you eat the same foods for meals and snacks as the rest of your family?
- What will this program cost you overall? Do you get a "deal" if you hit your goal? What about long-term membership options?
- Does this program have a maintenance program once weight loss is achieved?
- What type of professional support is available?

## Identifying Secrets to Successful Weight Loss

Most individuals seeking to lose weight are highly motivated by other successful dieters. Success stories and tips can help others when they may feel down about their past or current success. After speaking with many "who have been there," these "secrets" were compiled to help you get started, keep going, and to accomplish successful results.

- Take baby steps—one at a time.
- Eat small meals, up to five or six times per day, to avoid extreme hunger.
- Focus on lots of fruits and vegetables, high-fiber foods to help feel full.
- Set realistic goals.
- Don't think "diet"; think healthy eating.

- Always leave some food behind on your plate. If you are full, stop eating.
- Close the kitchen after 7:30 P.M.
- Keep moving, whatever it takes. Climb the stairs, walk the dog, or stay active during lunch: it all adds up.

Whatever route you take to lose weight, your primary goal is to educate yourself enough along the way so that you will be able to achieve self-sufficiency at some point down the road. You should eventually be able to manage your food intake, reduce your obsession with foods, and live a healthy lifestyle. Your basic goal in weight loss should be to make wise food choices while incorporating activity into your life. You need to learn to set realistic goals (both short- and long-term) and make a commitment to your health by losing slowly, safely, and effectively.

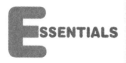**SSENTIALS**

Successful weight loss isn't about losing the weight and returning to old habits. It's about making a lifelong commitment to eating healthier and exercising regularly.

Remember, there is no magic answer. It is up to you to find out what works best for you. Keep yourself motivated, change your attitude, take one step at a time, and do it for your health.

CHAPTER 8

# Understanding Energy and Caloric Needs

I n the past several chapters, you began to curb your calorie intake based on reducing your total food intake. I told you about reducing total calories but offered suggestions through use of cutting back on food groups. Now it is time to elaborate on determining what your specific caloric needs are and how they are determined.

# What Is a Calorie?

To define a calorie, we would say that it is the amount of energy needed to raise the temperature of a gram of water by 1 degree Centigrade. So what does that mean? Calories (or the energy) in foods are measured by a scientific method called *direct calorimetry*. Through this process, foods are actually burned in a chamber surrounded by water to determine how many calories are contained within that particular food.

## Understanding Calorie Counts

Calorie counts are given to foods to show how much food energy they supply. Calorie counts are provided to consumers on nutrition labels found on food products as well as in many books and resources. People often become obsessed with calorie counts in the foods they eat, even without understanding the role calories provide in maintaining life and health.

**E**SSENTIALS

Protein, carbohydrates, and fats (and alcohol) are the only substances that contribute calories or energy to our diets.

Calories are terms that people are notorious for counting, tracking, eliminating, and discussing time and again because they are our most familiar measure of food. Calories are used to measure the amount of energy found in a food. The more calories a particular food has, the more energy it contains.

## Balancing Energy Needs

Energy gives us the ability to move, be active, and do work. By learning to understand energy needs, you can learn more about managing weight. Your goal should be to know what type of energy goes in and how that energy is used up. The energy in foods is measured and counted in calories. When the calories going in balance energy going out, body weight is maintained. When the calories going in exceed energy going out, body weight can be gained. And when the calories going in are less than energy going out, body weight can be lost.

# Where Do Calories Come From?

Three main groups of nutrients contribute calories to our diet: protein, carbohydrates, and fats. Protein and carbohydrates each contribute 4 calories per gram of food. Fat contributes 2½ times as many calories, at 9 calories per gram of food. Dietary recommendations suggest reducing fat in the diet primarily because fats are so highly concentrated in calories. (Alcohol is not considered a nutrient, but it also contributes calories to the diet at 7 calories per gram.)

Foods usually contain a combination of the calorie-contributing nutrients. These nutrients together contribute to that food's total caloric value. Let's look at several individual foods that you could opt for as a snack and see if that helps illustrate the contribution of calories from protein, carbohydrates, and fat.

One ounce of cheese snack-crackers has 3 grams of protein, 19 grams of carbohydrate, and 7 grams of fat. To determine how many calories the crackers have from protein, multiply the amount of protein (3 grams) times 4 calories/gram, and you see that it has 12 calories from protein. To determine how many calories the crackers get from carbohydrates, take the amount of carbohydrates (19 grams) and multiply it by 4 calories/gram to get 76 calories from carbohydrates. And to determine how many calories the crackers get from fat, multiply the amount of fat (7 grams) times 9 calories/gram to get 63 calories from fat. The total calorie count for the crackers is 151 calories per serving.

On the other hand, a ½ cup of low-fat cottage cheese has 12 grams of protein, 4 grams of carbohydrate, and 2 grams of fat. Multiply the 12 grams of protein times 4 calories/gram, and you see that the cottage cheese has 48 calories from protein. Multiply the 4 grams of carbohydrate times 4 calories/gram, and you see that it has 16 calories from carbohydrate. And multiply the 2 grams of fat times 9 calories/gram, and you get 18 calories from fat, for a total of 82 calories per serving.

We will examine nutrition labels in more detail in Chapter 16, but in the meantime these examples should help you understand a little more about where the caloric counts in foods actually come from. You can also determine further how determinations are made for total calories from fats and how fats can contribute excess calories to foods, thus adding excess calories to your diet.

## Determining Percentage of Fat

Look at the cheese crackers and cottage cheese again. Determine now what the percentage of fat is in a serving of these foods. To do so, divide the calories from fat by the total calories. So for the cheese crackers, divide 63 calories by 151 calories, and you see that 42 percent of the crackers' calories come from fat. For the cottage cheese, divide 18 calories by 82 calories, and you see that 21 percent of the calories come from fat.

You can see from these examples that almost half of the calories come from fat in the cheese snack-crackers, whereas only a fifth of the calories come from fat in the cottage cheese. Although either of these foods would be an adequate snack choice, the cottage cheese contributes a greater amount of protein and less fat than the snack crackers.

## Recommendation for Daily Calorie Intake

An overall healthy diet should include a combination of foods that contain protein, carbohydrates, and fats. The following breakdown demonstrates how each of these should contribute to the daily diet. By combining a variety of foods, you can meet this profile:

- Protein: 15 percent
- Carbohydrates: 55 percent (45 percent recommended as complex carbohydrates and no more than 10 percent from simple sugars)
- Fat: 30 percent (20 percent recommended as unsaturated fat and no more than 10 percent from saturated fat)

In actuality, the typical American diet is more like the following.

- Protein: 16 percent
- Carbohydrates: 50 percent
- Fat: 34 percent

Some improvements have been made in recent years, but further changes are necessary to help improve the nutritional status of the American population. Now let's examine the energy-producing nutrients in more detail.

# Carbohydrates: Your Primary Energy Source

Carbohydrates primarily include sugars and starches that come from plant sources, along with the natural sugar found in milk. These foods include simple sugars like sucrose (table sugar), fructose (fruit sugar), lactose (milk sugar), and maltose (malt sugar), and complex carbohydrates often referred to as starches. Starches are the carbohydrates of choice, as they contribute vitamins and minerals and are often lower in fat, lower in calories, and higher in fiber. Additionally, these complex carbohydrates help the body to maintain normal blood sugar (glucose) levels by promoting a slower, healthier digestion of foods in that starches take longer to digest than sugars. (This is one reason why competitive athletes are encouraged to eat a diet high in complex carbohydrate prior to competition and why individuals choosing to lose weight should also eat an abundance of these types of foods.)

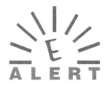

If your body doesn't have enough carbohydrates to use for energy, it will use protein (muscles, body tissues, and so on) for the energy that it needs.

## How Carbohydrates Are Used in the Body

All carbohydrates are broken down during digestion and converted to glucose (blood sugar), where they are then carried to body cells to be used for energy that the body needs. The pancreas then releases insulin to help move the glucose to the cells, where it is burned for energy. If there is more glucose than what the cells need, the remainder is stored in the muscles and liver as glycogen and reserved for later use. If the glycogen stores are full and there is still more glucose, it is then stored as fat. Any amount over and above what the body needs is converted to body fat.

## Carbohydrates and Weight Reduction

Many people believe that carbohydrates are taboo when it comes to weight reducing. This is a total myth. Carbohydrates only become a problem with weight gain when too many are consumed, when the wrong type is consumed, or when preparation methods add excess amounts of fats, like covering pasta (a healthy complex carbohydrate choice) with excess amounts of cream sauce (a not-so-healthy higher-fat choice). Rice with butter, mashed potatoes with gravy, and a bagel with cream cheese are also similar examples of adding fat to a healthy complex carbohydrate food.

Carbohydrates, especially complex carbohydrates, are actually the food of choice when seeking to reduce body weight. These foods are highly nutritious, low in fat, and high in fiber.

## Contribution of Carbohydrates to the Overall Diet

Carbohydrates should contribute at least 55 percent of the total calories in the diet. For a person consuming a 2,000-calorie diet, that would equate to 1,100 total calories from carbohydrates. Vegetables, fruits, and grains, like breads, pasta, rice, and cereals, are high in carbohydrates. Legumes (dried beans and peas) are excellent sources as well.

# Protein: The Body's Building Blocks

Protein is not the body's energy source of choice, but it can be used for energy when there are not enough carbohydrates and fats in the diet. The protein you consume contributes to the development of muscles, bones, cartilage, skin, antibodies, hormones, and enzymes in your body. It is important in the building and maintaining of all bodily structures.

## How Protein Is Used in the Body

Protein is built by a combination of chemical structures called *amino acids*. There are about twenty amino acids that the body needs, and these are often referred to as the building blocks of body. Of the twenty amino acids, nine are essential to the diet, meaning they must be supplied by the foods we eat. The remaining amino acids can be made in the body. When a food is consumed that includes all nine of the essential amino acids, it is referred to as a complete protein source. Meat, poultry, fish, eggs, and dairy products like milk and cheese all are complete protein sources. Incomplete sources of protein are those that do not contain the amount of essential amino acids needed by the body. These sources are primarily those fruits and vegetables. But some plant sources offer some of the essential amino acids while others offer the remaining ones. By combining various sources of plant proteins with each other, a complete protein source can be made. For example, if rice is consumed with beans, this combination becomes a complete protein source. These combinations of foods are necessary for vegetarians who do not eat meat sources of protein and may have difficulties in meeting protein requirements. More can be found on vegetarianism in Chapter 11.

FACTS

Your body needs the right balance of all twenty amino acids in order to adequately build tissues in the body. If any one is missing, the protein will not be built.

## Protein Requirements

The amount of protein needed by a person is based on age, sex, and body size. The Recommended Dietary Allowance for protein in adult males over twenty years of age ranges from 58 to 63 grams per day. For adult females over twenty, the allowance ranges from 46 to 50 grams per day. Most people do not have trouble meeting protein requirements. In fact, many often consume more than they need, up to twice as much.

## Protein and Weight Reduction

Many people have been drawn to weight-reduction diets that are high in protein. Individuals have found that these high-protein diets actually lead to weight loss. But excess protein in the diet is not a wise choice. Too much protein (any in many cases too much fat that results as well) can lead to risk of health problems along with a condition called *ketosis*. This condition develops from not having significant sources of energy (from carbohydrates) that, as a result, makes the body use protein for energy. It can cause extra work for the liver and kidneys and can actually be harmful in the long run. This is one reason that consuming excess protein through high-protein diets is not a healthy way to lose weight.

## Contribution of Protein to the Overall Diet

Protein should account for about 15 percent of total daily calories. For a person consuming a 2,000-calorie diet, this would equate to about 300 total calories. A variety of lean meats, poultry, fish, eggs, low-fat dairy products, and dried beans and peas should contribute to this intake.

# Fat: An Essential Nutrient

Many people believe all fats are bad for our diet. Too much fat is linked to health problems like heart disease, stroke, obesity, and some types of cancers. But, in fact, fats are an essential part of all cells in the body. Fat helps maintain the health of the skin and hair, transports fat-soluble vitamins (vitamins A, D, E, K) throughout the body, cushions the body organs to keep them safe from injury, and serves as a protective insulator to the body on cold days. In addition, fats contribute to the taste, smell, and texture of foods as well as providing a satiety factor of fullness after eating foods that contain it. The reason fats take so long to digest is because they are so calorie dense, containing 2½ times the amount of calories that are found in carbohydrates and protein. But in order to meet your body's need for fat, you should aim to eat foods with the right type and amount of fat.

## The Various Types of Fat

Understanding fats can be confusing. We often hear about saturated, unsaturated, and polyunsaturated fats. The differences between these types of fats are a result of their chemical makeup. The more hydrogen the chemical makeup contains, the more saturated the fat becomes. It is also possible to distinguish some fats by their appearance. Saturated fats are those that are typically solid at room temperature, like lard, butterfat, and beef fat (the fat marbled throughout meat).

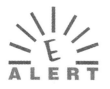
**ALERT**

Don't be fooled by coconut oil, palm oil, and palm kernel oil. These fats may be liquid, but they are actually saturated fats, the kind that can increase health risks of heart disease and cancer.

Health risks are primarily associated with diets high in saturated fats and are known to increase overall risk of heart disease and some types of cancer. Unsaturated and polyunsaturated fats are usually from plant sources and are liquid or soft at room temperature. These examples include oils like corn, olive, canola, peanut, soybean, sunflower, and safflower oils. These fats can actually help decrease health-related problems and reduce risk factors of heart disease and various types of cancers. Several exceptions to the rule include the tropical oils of coconut oil, palm oil, and palm kernel oil. Although these are vegetable oils and liquid at room temperature, these actually fall into the category of saturated fats.

## Cholesterol

Cholesterol is not a fat but often categorized with fats. It is a white, waxy type of fat substance found in animal products. It is an important component in the diet in the building of tissue and cell walls, and it is required for the manufacture of hormones and bile. Cholesterol, a component of many foods like butter, egg yolk, meat fat, poultry skin, organ meats, and shellfish, is also made in the body. Because of health concerns with excessive consumption, cholesterol should be limited to 300 milligrams or less per day.

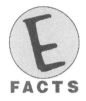

**FACTS**

Cholesterol is found only in animal tissues. Therefore, foods containing it must come from an animal source. Foods like peanut butter cannot contain cholesterol.

## Fat Requirements

Fat is essential to the diet early in life as it contributes to brain development and the building of the spine and central nervous system. The first two years of a person's life are considered crucial, with recommendations that over 50 percent of the diet should come from fat during the first year alone. This drops off slightly during the second year of life. After this time, children—just like adults—should consume no more than 30 percent of their total daily calories from fat. Some researchers and resources suggest decreasing fat intake to as little as 20 percent of daily calories, but studies have indicated that too little fat can actually be more harmful to the body.

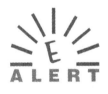

**ALERT**

To prevent problems associated with heart attacks, stroke, and certain types of cancer, individuals should aim for no more than 30 percent of their daily intake from fat.

## Fat and Weight Control

For most Americans, cutting back to 30 percent of total calories from fat is a suggested goal, with 10 percent or less of this total coming from saturated fat. But it is not necessary to track the percentage of every kind of fat you eat. Instead, a simpler method would be to watch those fat grams. A diet that combines a variety of foods, both higher and lower in fat, in moderate portions helps to provide the variety and balance you need. Refer back to the chart on page 63 (Chapter 5) to help you determine your daily fat requirement.

# How Many Calories Do You Need?

Although it is not necessary to be totally focused on a specific caloric requirement, it is helpful to understand approximately how many calories it takes for your body to function. This will, in turn, help you to estimate how much you need to reduce your intake of foods in order to lose the weight you want.

## Resting Metabolic Needs

To get a general idea of the number of calories you need to lose weight, you first need to estimate the number of calories you need to maintain your body weight—your body weight at its current level. In doing so you first must establish how many calories it takes to maintain your normal body functions at rest. This is referred to as your basal metabolic rate (BMR). Once you determine this number, then you will be able to add additional calories to compensate for daily activities and needs for basic body functions. I'll show you how. Start with this equation:

To determine your BMR, multiply your current weight by ten (for women) or eleven (for men). A 150-pound woman has a BMR of 1,500. This is the approximate amount of energy (calories) that this individual needs at rest. (Although BMR is primarily calculated from kilogram weight, this formula will still provide you with an accurate estimate of your needs without converting weight to kilograms.)

## Activity Needs

But because people do more than just rest, and because our bodies need energy (calories) to meet physical needs, we must further determine our activity needs.

To determine your activity needs do the following.

- If you are mostly sedentary during the day (sitting, standing, reading, writing, and not doing much physical activity), multiply your BMR by 0.20.
- If you are lightly active during the day (doing housework, playing with children, walking two miles or less during the course of the day), multiply your BMR by 0.30.
- If you are somewhat active during the day (doing heavy housework or gardening, playing tennis, working out at a club, dancing), multiply your BMR by 0.40.
- If you are very active during the day (working in construction, doing heavy labor, playing team sports regularly), multiply your BMR by 0.50.

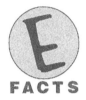

**FACTS**

Metabolism is defined as all the work your body does that uses calories—the work needed to stay alive, think, breathe, and move.

So our lightly active 150-pound woman, with a BMR of 1,500, would multiply 1,500 times 0.30. Her adjustment for activity needs would be 450. That mean she needs 1,500 calories just to get by without any physical activity, but she needs another 450 calories on top of that to accommodate her activity. Her total BMR would be 1,500 plus 450, or 1,950 calories.

## Basic Digestive/Absorption Needs

A final factor must be taken into account for those energy requirements for basic digestive functions. This factor includes needs for basic bodily functions like digesting food and absorbing nutrients in the body. This will account for about 10 percent of your daily calories. Take your total BMR (with activity factored in) times 0.10. So the woman from the last section, with a total BMR of 1,950, would multiply 1,950 by 0.10, to get 195. Add that to 1,950, and you see she needs 2,145 calories to maintain her current weight.

This formula is just a guideline for people to determine their approximate BMR. There are many factors that contribute to it as well. Outside of differences that exist between men and women, BMR is also affected by heredity and body composition.

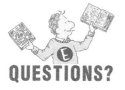

**How does your basal metabolic rate add up?**
Your BMR is a result of your daily basal metabolic needs (about 60 to 70 percent), your daily activity needs (about 20 to 30 percent), and your daily digestion/absorption needs (about 10 percent).

# Understanding Nutrition and Weight Loss

Fast or slow metabolisms can become inherited. (Wouldn't we all love to have a fast metabolism?) This is why some people stay thin throughout their life while eating whatever they desire, while others feel like the pounds just pile on. Your body composition is also a factor in determining your BMR. Some people's bodies have more muscle, others more bone, while yet others have more fat. A person who is muscular and lean will have a higher metabolism than someone built with a larger amount of fat. Muscle burns more energy (calories) than fat does. So the more muscle you have, the more calories you will burn. This is why it is so important to build those muscles throughout life. You can do this by adopting a strength-training program in addition to planned cardiovascular activity. (You can find more about this in Chapter 14.)

## Differences Between Men and Women

Of course, women are also prone to burning fewer calories than men are. This is a fact. This is because a woman's body contains a higher percentage of fat than a man's body. Men usually have 10 to 20 percent more muscle than women do, and they therefore burn calories at a higher rate. Women's bodies have increased fat stores to help them compensate during times of special needs during their lives, like during pregnancy and lactation.

## Losing One Pound at a Time

Now let's determine how many calories are necessary to begin to lose weight in a healthy manner. As stated in the last chapter, 3,500 calories equal 1 pound. To lose 1 pound you will need to decrease your caloric intake by 3,500 calories. You can see from the above example that it is not possible to put your body in a deficit of 3,500 calories within the course of a day or two. But you can decrease your calories sufficiently by 500 calories per day to lose 1 pound per week (500 calories multiplied by seven days equals 3,500 calories). You need to create a negative energy balance—consume fewer calories than you use up without sacrificing your other nutrient needs. This will allow for a weight loss of about 1 pound per week.

Initially this may seem too low for you. You are much more interested in losing at a faster rate than this. But as we have previously discussed, this approach will help you to lose body fat (not muscle or water weight), incorporate a healthier food intake, and achieve permanent results.

Let's look back at our earlier example. Our 150-pound woman needs 2,145 calories to maintain her weight. To lose weight effectively and efficiently, a deficit of 500 calories per day would allow her to consume 1,645 calories per day for an average weight loss of 1 pound per week. This weight loss would be slow and adequate, while the calorie allotment would allow for balanced meals and snack options throughout three meals and several snacks during the day.

As you begin to lose weight, you can also increase your activity levels to burn even more calories. This will help bring on a larger deficit of calories, thus helping to lose at a slightly higher rate.

## The Connection Between Age and Decreasing Metabolism

As people age, their metabolism declines. Each decade (after twenty-five to thirty years of age) results in an energy decline of somewhere between 3 to 5 percent. The reason the metabolism decreases is because our bodies change over the years. Body composition changes. Hormones cause changes. Bodies become less active. Muscle tissue declines. Body fat increases. Because there is less muscle mass overall, fewer calories are burned for normal energy needs, thus resulting in a metabolic decline.

For example, our 150-pound woman who requires 2,145 calories to maintain her weight at thirty years of age will need about 2,100 calories at age forty and closer to 2,000 calories at age fifty. Exercise and physical activity throughout life, particularly strength training, can help counterbalance this decline because they help increase muscle tissue thus accelerating metabolism and calorie needs. Just working out your major muscle groups twice each week can help replace a decade's loss of muscle mass in several months. Lifting weights and building strength helps reduce the aging process and makes you feel younger and stronger along the way.

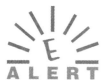

Unless exercise is incorporated into regular lifestyles, a person's metabolism can decrease as much as 3 to 5 percent each decade during adult life.

## Reasons for Weight Gain

People over twenty-five and up to sixty-five years of age often experience weight gain. Some attribute this to aging and, indeed, that is a factor. But aging isn't just to blame. When people first begin their professional careers just after high school or college and up until the retirement years, they often become more sedentary. Weight gain can creep up here and there until a few pounds turn into an overweight or obese condition. As lifestyles become more affluent, so do higher standards of living, requiring less labor overall. When people hire help to clean their houses, cut their grass, or wash their cars, they save themselves the work and burn fewer calories, too. People also take advantage of various eating opportunities, choosing to eat out more often, enjoying social eating events, and spending more money on food overall. Each one of these can contribute to weight gain over the years.

## Do People Have a Predetermined Weight?

You may notice over the years that some people can maintain their weight without a great deal of effort while others fight to lose beyond a certain point. Many nutrition scientists believe in a theory, often referred to as the *set point theory*.

A set point is a weight range that your body aims to maintain. It is programmed for you based on your genetic and chemical makeup. Your body works hard to stay within a minimal range surrounding this set point. The body's metabolism decreases when weight drops lower than its set point so weight loss is slow; on the contrary, it increases when weight rises above the set point. The body works hard to keep this balance. Set points are often noticed when comparing two people of the size height and same frame size. Even if these two people ate the same foods, they would not necessarily gain weight the same way or lose weight the same way. The weight they carry is dependent on their genetic makeup and ultimately on their set point. The set point theory can explain many mysteries surrounding weight reduction and dieting.

As we can see from this information in this chapter, every person's energy needs are different. Various factors contribute to the differences. Although it may be helpful to determine your particular needs, doing so will just help you estimate a guideline within which to work. Body size, metabolism, age, gender, activity levels, and genetics all are factors in determining one's exact energy needs. Rather than focusing on a specific number, individuals should try to understand where energy comes from and how they can aim to properly meet individual food energy requirements. This can be much more effective in losing and maintaining overall weight. By doing so you can also work on creating a plan toward a healthier lifestyle.

CHAPTER 9

# The Noncaloric Nutrients: Vitamins, Minerals, and Water

Vitamins and minerals are essential nutrients that are widely spread throughout our food supply. They are extremely necessary to overall health. Whenever changes are made to your diet, care must be taken to assure proper balance and intake of the essential nutrients. Here you will learn more about why.

## Vitamins: The Organic Compounds

Vitamins are organic compounds that are essential to health. Vitamins are not made by the body (although in some cases, one form can be made into another within the body) and must be supplied by the foods we eat. But unlike protein, carbohydrates, and fats, vitamins provide no energy source.

Vitamins are essential to life. Each vitamin has known functions in the body. But only small amounts are required. Daily requirements of all the vitamins combined would add up to only about $\frac{1}{8}$ teaspoon. But even with requirements so small, vitamins are necessary to support life. Without the required amount of a particular vitamin, deficiency symptoms could develop. Not after a day or two of missing an intake, but in the course of several months or more, each has been shown to develop signs of deficiency, though very few cases of known vitamin deficiencies occur in the United States. Vitamins are clearly divided into two main groups: fat-soluble and water-soluble vitamins.

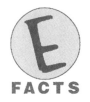

**FACTS**

Vitamins and minerals are as important to the diet as the energy-producing nutrients, protein, carbohydrates, and fats, only they do not supply calories and do not supply energy. Instead, vitamins and minerals are the key to many processes and activities that occur inside our bodies everyday. Because of this, these nutrients need to be supplied in adequate amounts each day.

## Fat-Soluble Vitamins

The fat-soluble vitamins are vitamins A, D, E, and K. These vitamins have the ability to be stored in the body if excesses are consumed. This can be a benefit to many people who do not consume adequate amounts each day. Unfortunately for others, toxic levels can occur if too large amounts are consumed over time. Toxic levels can become dangerous to the body. Let's focus in on these important vitamins, what they do, and what food sources supply them.

## Vitamin A

Vitamin A exists in two forms. Foods of animal origin provide vitamin A, the active form of the vitamin, whereas foods from plant sources provide a provitamin type, referred to as *beta-carotene*, that converts to vitamin A in the body. Vitamin A is supplied in foods like liver, fish oils, fortified dairy products, and egg yolks. Beta-carotene is found in foods like carrots, sweet potatoes, pumpkin, spinach, broccoli, squash, peppers, papaya, mango, cantaloupe, and apricots. Foods high in beta-carotene are also beneficial as antioxidants, meaning they provide protective benefits to preventing disease and tissue damage.

Vitamin A is necessary for building bones and healthy epithelial tissue, the tissue found in the skin, eyes, and the passages of the lungs, intestines, and reproductive organs. Vitamin A is known for keeping skin and hair healthy. It is also needed to maintain healthy eyesight, especially at night and in dim lighting conditions.

## Vitamin D

Vitamin D is a unique vitamin in that it can be supplied from foods in the diet or from direct exposure to the sun. Necessary to help regulate calcium levels in the bloodstream, this vitamin plays an important role in building strong bones and teeth. Vitamin D can be found in some fish (sardines and salmon) and fish oils, cheese, eggs, butter, and fortified milk, cereal, and margarine products.

FACTS

Vitamin D is often referred to as the "sunshine vitamin" because it can be supplied by exposure to the sun. People who live in sunny climates should have no difficulties in obtaining their requirement of vitamin D.

## Vitamin E

Vitamin E is a well-known vitamin in that it is highly promoted as a cure-all to many people. Although many claims to this are unsubstantiated, this vitamin has gained popularity in recent years. Essential in maintaining a healthy immune and nervous system, vitamin E is also known to provide antioxidant effects to help protect against tissue damage and disease. A diet with foods rich in vitamin E includes vegetable oils, like soybean, corn, safflower, and cottonseed, margarine, some fruits and vegetables, wheat germ, multigrain cereals, nuts and seeds.

## Vitamin K

The main function of vitamin K is to contribute to blood clotting. This vitamin is needed to make proteins that help clot the blood in the event of a cut, scrape, or bleeding injury. Vitamin K is supplied by a varied diet consisting of dark green leafy vegetables, liver, fruits, milk, meats, eggs, and grain products.

# Water-Soluble Vitamins

Water-soluble vitamins (B-complex and vitamin C, also known as ascorbic acid) are not stored in the body. In fact, these vitamins dissolve in water, so if excesses are consumed, they are usually excreted in the urine. These vitamins cannot build up excess amounts in the body. But, as a result, these vitamins need to be consumed on a daily basis in order to obtain recommended amounts. These vitamins are widely available in many food sources.

## Thiamin (B-1)

Thiamin plays an important role in energy metabolism. It is also required for functions of the nerves and muscles. Thiamin can be found in whole-grain breads and cereals, pork products, liver, dried beans, nuts and seeds, as well as in enriched products to which the vitamin has been added after refining.

## Riboflavin (B$_2$)

Riboflavin assists the body in releasing energy from carbohydrates, fats, and proteins. Primary sources of riboflavin are milk and milk products, but enriched and whole-grain cereals, organ meat (such as liver, kidney, or heart), meats, poultry, eggs, fish, dark green leafy vegetables, and nuts also provide this vitamin.

## Niacin

Niacin is mainly involved in energy metabolism, but it assists in keeping the skin and nervous system healthy as well. Whole-grain and enriched breads and cereals as well as meats, poultry, fish, peanut butter, legumes, and nuts are main sources of this vitamin.

What is the difference between a food that has been fortified and one that has been enriched? Fortified means that one or more nutrients have been added to a food during processing. Prior to processing these nutrients were not found in the food, as in fortifying milk with vitamin D. On the contrary, enriching a food means to add vitamins and minerals back to the food after the nutrients have been lost during the refining process.

## Pantothenic Acid

This vitamin plays an important role in energy metabolism, but it also promotes growth as well. It can be found in a variety of food sources, including meats, poultry, fish, whole-grain breads and cereals, legumes, milk, fruits, and vegetables.

## Biotin

Biotin helps produce energy from carbohydrates, proteins, and fats. It is found in egg yolks, yeast, cereals, liver, cheese, and nuts.

## Vitamin B$_6$

Vitamin B$_6$ plays an essential role in the metabolism of fats and in helping build body tissues. Its food sources include meats, fish, poultry, pork, organ meats, dairy products, whole grains, and some fruits and vegetables, like bananas, cantaloupe, broccoli, and spinach.

## Folate (Folic Acid)

Important particularly to women of childbearing age, this vitamin assists in developing new cells in the body and in synthesizing DNA (the genetic makeup of the cells). Dark green leafy vegetables are a main source of this vitamin, along with liver, yeast, wheat germ, legumes, oranges, cantaloupe, and broccoli. Enriched breads and cereal products also supply adequate amounts of folate.

## Vitamin $B_{12}$ (Cobalamin)

Vitamin $B_{12}$ helps folate function. It also is necessary for growth and maintenance of healthy nerve tissue and the formation of red blood cells. Because it is primarily found in meat, poultry, fish, eggs, and dairy products, this vitamin is often a concern of vegetarians. Strict vegetarians who do not eat any meat, eggs, fish, or dairy products must often seek alternative sources of vitamin $B_{12}$.

## Vitamin C (Ascorbic Acid)

A well-known vitamin, vitamin C performs a number of important functions within the body. It helps in the formation of collagen, which holds the cells together that are necessary for healthy bones, cartilage, muscles, and blood vessels; assists in wound healing; increases the absorption of iron and calcium; serves as an antioxidant in preventing cell damage; and protects against illness and disease.

Vitamin C is abundant in fruits and many vegetables including citrus fruits, cantaloupe, strawberries, broccoli, potatoes, tomatoes, cabbage, dark green leafy vegetables (such as romaine lettuce, spinach, turnip greens), and green and red peppers.

# Minerals: The Inorganic Elements

Like vitamins, minerals are nutrients that the body needs in extremely small amounts. They, too, provide no calories. But unlike vitamins, minerals are inorganic elements, meaning they are not compounds, and they do not contain carbon.

There are at least sixteen different types of minerals that are important in the diet. These can fall into the categories of macrominerals and microminerals. Each type is equally important; the body simply requires them in different amounts. Recommended daily requirements of minerals are extremely small, but they are very important to good health. Minerals, in general, help enzymes complete chemical reactions, aid in normal nerve functions and muscle contraction, promote growth, regulate acid-base balance, and maintain body fluid balance.

# Macrominerals

Macrominerals include calcium, phosphorus, magnesium, sulfur, potassium, and chloride. These may be more familiar to most people in that they are required in somewhat larger amounts than the micronutrients. Let's focus in on each of these popular minerals.

## Calcium

Calcium is the mineral found in greatest amounts within the body and rightfully so. It is largely found in the bones to help maintain bone mass and strengthen bones throughout life. Additionally, calcium is used to build strong teeth. It is important for muscle contraction, the beating of the heart, nerve functioning, and blood clotting. The dairy group offers the greatest amount of calcium to the diet, although dark green leafy vegetables, legumes, and sardines supply calcium as well. Many foods today are also fortified with calcium, like orange juice.

## Phosphorus

Phosphorus and calcium work together in the body to help form strong bones and teeth. Phosphorus also helps in regulating energy metabolism. It can be found in almost all foods that are rich in protein, like milk, poultry, cheese, meats, legumes, eggs, and nuts, and also in breads, potatoes, peas, raisins, and avocados.

## Magnesium

Like calcium and phosphorus, much of the body's magnesium is also found in the bones. Primarily, magnesium serves the body by making enzymes active so they can work more efficiently. It is also helpful for the lungs, nerves, and functions of the heart. Food sources of magnesium include dark green leafy vegetables, potatoes, legumes, seafood, nuts, dairy foods, and whole grains.

## Sulfur

Sulfur is found in every body cell. It helps maintain the acid-base balance in the body. In addition, sulfur helps the liver transform toxins in the body into less harmful substances. Since the body needs sulfur in extremely small amounts, no dietary requirements exists, although sulfur is found in protein-rich foods and those that contain the B-vitamins thiamin and biotin.

## Sodium, Potassium, Chloride

These three minerals work together to help regulate fluid balance in the body. Although sodium occurs naturally in many foods, its primary contribution comes from table salt and processed foods. Table salt, also known as sodium chloride, also supplies chloride to the diet. Potassium is found in fresh fruits and vegetables, milk, meat, poultry, and various types of fish.

# Microminerals

The microminerals are extremely important in body functions even though they are needed only in very small amounts. Following is a rundown of these essential nutrients.

## Iron

Iron is one of the most important minerals in the body, which is mostly found within the blood. Iron is part of the hemoglobin, a protein that helps red blood cells transport oxygen from the lungs to the cells. Hemoglobin also carries carbon dioxide from the body tissues back to the lungs for excretion. Because iron is part of the blood cells, it can be depleted if blood stores are depleted. As a result, too little iron in the body can result in a condition referred to as anemia, a type of iron deficiency. This makes the blood less able to carry oxygen, causing tiredness, fatigue, and loss of appetite. Iron-rich foods should be a part of everyone's diet. These include red meat, clams, oysters, duck, dark green leafy vegetables, and enriched whole grains and cereals. Iron is also more highly absorbed by the body when consumed with food rich in vitamin C, for example when an iron-enriched cereal is eaten along with a glass of orange juice.

## Zinc

Zinc contributes to numerous body functions, including growth and sexual development. It also helps increase enzyme functions. Additionally it helps with acid-base balance and helps the body resist infections. Zinc can be found in foods like red meats, seafood, liver, eggs, milk, whole grains, wheat germ, legumes, and nuts.

## Iodine

Iodine plays a role in metabolic functions within the body, particularly in producing a hormone called *thyroxine*, which controls metabolism. Iodine is mostly found in saltwater fish and iodized salt (table salt with added iodine).

## Fluoride

Fluoride is commonly thought of in connection to water as it occurs naturally in some water and is added to other water sources. Fluoride is important for healthy bones and teeth. Outside of the water supply, it can be found in tea and in fish (like canned salmon) that have edible bones.

## Selenium

Selenium works as an antioxidant in conjunction with vitamin E. It is also responsible for maintaining cell growth. Selenium can mostly be found in meats, liver, eggs, fish, and shellfish.

## Copper, Chromium, Manganese, Molybdenum

Each of these minerals also benefits body processes. Copper helps make hemoglobin and contributes to keeping bones, blood vessels, and nerves healthy. It is found in beans, seeds, seafood, nuts, seeds, and organ meats. Chromium aids in glucose metabolism and can be found in egg yolks, meats, cheese, mushrooms, nuts, and yeast. Manganese plays a role in carbohydrate metabolism and enzyme functions. It is available in whole grains, beans, and dark green leafy vegetables. And molybdenum plays a role in enzyme activity and is found in dairy foods, nuts, beans, and whole-grain products.

# Phytonutrients

Phytonutrients, also referred to as *phytochemicals*, are not vitamins or minerals per se but compounds found in various foods that appear to fight diseases like heart disease, various types of cancers, eye disorders, and problems with blood clots. These chemical compounds are also noted for giving fruits and vegetables their many vibrant colors. By choosing a variety of colorful fruits and vegetables each day, you can obtain the greatest amount of disease-fighting substances in the diet.

Various names attributed to these compounds include:

- Lycopene
- Flavonoids
- Alpha-beta carotene
- Cryptoxanthin

- Lutein
- Zeaxanthin
- Antioxidants

Try these colorful selections in your foods:

- **Red:** Tomatoes, watermelons, guava, pink grapefruit
- **Dark red/purple:** Grapes, grape juice, blackberries, cranberries, apples, prunes, strawberries, eggplant, plums
- **Orange:** Sweet potatoes, mangoes, carrots, apricots, cantaloupe, pumpkin
- **Orange/yellow:** Oranges, tangerines, clementines, peaches, papayas, nectarines
- **Yellow/green:** Corn, avocado, peaches, honeydew
- **Green:** Brussels sprouts, broccoli, green beans, peas, spinach, romaine, kale
- **White/green:** Garlic, onions, chives
- **Blue:** Blueberries

Vitamins and minerals are widely found in our food supply. They can be healthfully obtained by consuming a diet rich in protein, fruits, vegetables, dairy products, and grains. In other words, an adequate vitamin supply comes from a diet that contains all the food groups. But many people are not satisfied with their wide availability. Many people continually seek alternative methods to supply themselves with these nutrients.

# Are Vitamin and Mineral Supplements Necessary?

People spend billions and billions of dollars yearly on supplements of all types. Once referred to simply as vitamin supplements, these supplements are now in pill, capsule, powder, or liquid form. They include vitamins and minerals as well as herbs, botanicals, fiber, amino acids, and other extracts. Many people choose to take these supplements because they worry that they just don't eat enough of the right kinds of foods, kind of like an "insurance policy" for nutrients. Others do so for protective benefits, thinking more is better in the fight against illness and disease. And still others do so as a "miracle cure," thinking that a supplement may cure or eliminate a health problem. Are these dollars being spent wisely? Are all these supplements really necessary?

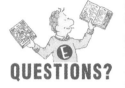

**QUESTIONS?**

**Are natural or synthetic vitamin/mineral supplements a better choice?**
Chemically speaking, neither offers any benefits over the other. Both natural and synthetic supplements work the same within the body. Your body cannot distinguish between the two types.

Vitamin/mineral supplements are just that, a "supplement." They are not "miracle cures," do not enhance energy, and do not make up for poor nutrition. The only thing that they can do is to provide the vitamin or mineral source in question and help prevent its deficiency.

Recommended dietary allowances of each vitamin and mineral are available for consumers to understand how much of each source is necessary on a daily basis. Many supplements offer much more than these recommended levels. For the water-soluble vitamins, this may present no immediate problems as excesses are eliminated in the urine. But in the case of fat-soluble vitamins, excesses are stored and can become toxic if levels become excessive. Always check dosages before taking any product and do not take excessive levels of any vitamin or mineral unless otherwise prescribed by your doctor.

Supplements can be costly. They provide no energy or fuel, no fiber, no taste, and no satiety. They provide none of the benefits you find in the wide variety of foods available. Wouldn't you agree that getting these vitamins and minerals from the foods we eat is much more beneficial?

In some instances, however, supplements may be necessary. A physician may prescribed vitamin supplements when needs are greater, as in the case of an illness, a chronic condition, or pregnancy, or under special conditions like breastfeeding or during recovery from surgery.

Supplements may also be required for those following strict vegetarian diets or for individuals who may get little exposure to the sun. But in most cases, a diet that includes foods from all the major food groups in moderate portions should be adequate to meet recommended vitamin and mineral needs.

# What about Water?

Water is an essential nutrient, just like protein, carbohydrates, fats, vitamins, and minerals. It plays a vital role in health and is quite necessary for survival. In fact, without water a person could only survive for several days; without food, a person could last much longer.

> Without water in the diet, a person could only survive for a few days. On the contrary, depending on a person's state of health, their survival without food could last eight to ten weeks.

Water is a part of every body cell. It is a large part of the body, in as much as 50 to 70 percent of one's total body weight. Body fluids, like blood, saliva, digestive juices, urine, and perspiration primarily consist of water. Water benefits the body by assisting in chemical reactions, carrying nutrients to the cells, helping remove waste products, controlling body temperature, and keeping body fluids balanced.

## Water Requirements

In order for your body to maintain its body fluids and keep them healthy, it is important for you to obtain an adequate intake of water each day. Six to eight glasses of water are recommended daily as a fluid intake. This is an adequate amount to replace lost body fluids. This can come from water itself or from the foods you eat. Milk, juices, soups, and other liquids contribute to this overall total, as well as foods with a high water content, like fruits and vegetables.

## Water and Weight Reduction

As mentioned earlier, water weight is often a concern in weight loss. Because your body is highly composed of water, when you aim to lose some weight, you will often lose body fluids as well—especially with restrictive weight-loss diets. But water weight is quickly regained once diet and fluid requirements are again met. Water weight is not the same as fat weight. Although numbers may change temporarily on the scale, this is not the way to reduce healthfully. In fact, too much water loss can result in dehydration, a state in which the body is too low in fluids, which can cause health problems and malfunctioning of body organs.

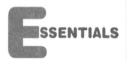

For best control of your body fluids, respond to your thirst. Drink water when you're thirsty. It is refreshing, and it's the healthiest fluid replacement for your body.

Vitamins, minerals, and water are all essential to health and well-being. You can see how each of these nutrients contributes in its own way to the inner workings of the body. Without the required amounts, the body cannot function properly. Whether you are aiming to maintain or lose weight, all of these nutrients are vital to your success. Keep this in mind as you plan your daily meals and snacks.

CHAPTER 10

# The World of Sugar and Fat Substitutes

**W**ouldn't it be wonderful if we could take all those excess sugars and fats out of the foods we eat, and be able to eat anything and everything we want, without any of the consequences? Some people believe we can. But as you read on, you may again realize that some things sound just too good to be true.

# Cutting the Sugar out of Food

We start with sugar substitutes. These are replacements for sugar that taste very similar to table sugar (sucrose) but that are, in fact, much, much sweeter. Many of these sweeteners supply no calories. Others supply only a minimal number of calories, thus creating foods with substantially reduced total calories.

# Types of Sugar Substitutes

Sugar substitutes, also referred to as artificial sweeteners, are likely to be found in diet soft drinks, puddings, baked goods, yogurt, and chewing gum. They can also be used as a tabletop sweetener.

Because of the way these types of products decrease excess sugar and the total calories people consume, the demand for sugar substitutes has skyrocketed in recent years. But, instead of consuming less sweetener overall, people are now using more than three times the amount of artificial sweeteners they used only a decade ago.

ALERT

A regular 12-ounce can of soft drink contains upwards of 10 teaspoons of sugar and 100 calories and can be compared to the same size diet soft drink at 0 teaspoons of sugar and 0 calories.

## Do You Remember Cyclamate?

You may remember back in the 1950s when cyclamates were a commonly used sugar substitute in this country. Heat stable and at least thirty times as sweet as sugar, this sweetener became very popular and was included in foods like baked goods, cereal, canned goods, beverages, toothpaste, and even mouthwash. But years later, in the late 1960s, cyclamate was shown to have caused bladder tumors in laboratory rats that were fed large doses of the sweetener. Following these results, the FDA banned cyclamate from use in our country.

More studies have been conducted since this time and have shown no evidence that this sweetener is carcinogenic, but it has yet to be reapproved for use. Cyclamate remains approved outside the United States. It continues to be used in Canada and more than fifty other countries, including Europe, Asia, South America, and Africa.

**E**SSENTIALS   Sugar substitutes that replace sugar in foods and as tabletop sweeteners can be up to 2,000 times as sweet as sugar itself.

## Saccharin

Saccharin, frequently known as Sweet & Low or the "pink sugar," then became the sugar sweetener of choice. Being 300 times as sweet as sugar, this popular sugar substitute has been used for years in many baked products, beverages, soft drinks, and as a tabletop sweetener. Controversies soon began arising about the safety of saccharin as well because it had been shown to cause cancer in laboratory animals but not in humans. But no substantiated data indicated the need to remove this sweetener from the market. Instead, products were required to be labeled (since 1977) indicating that the food product contained saccharin, a substance that had been shown to develop bladder cancer in laboratory animals. Only recently has this labeling requirement been eliminated.

## Aspartame

In 1981, after more than a decade of extensive safety testing, the Food and Drug Administration approved another sugar substitute. Known as *aspartame*, this sweetener is marketed under the names NutraSweet and Equal. It is comprised of two amino acids (aspartic acid and phenylalanine). Aspartame tastes very similar to sugar itself, offers 200 times its sweetness, and has no caloric value. Many products contain aspartame, like baked goods, canned foods, puddings, gelatins, frozen desserts, beverage mixes, hot cocoa, diet soft drinks, and chewing gum. It is not heat stable, so products using aspartame must be ones that do not require much cooking or baking. NutraSweet (Equal) is also available as a tabletop sweetener, packaged in blue and available for adding to beverages like coffee and tea and to be sprinkled over the top of cereal and yogurt.

Controversies regarding the use of this sugar substitute arose, and safety testing continued, but no research has yet indicated that this sweetener is unsafe, especially when used in moderate portions. Guidelines set by the FDA for aspartame use far exceed the amounts commonly consumed by most people.

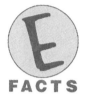

**FACTS**

An average-sized adult would have to consume more than fifteen (12-ounce) cans of diet soft drink made with aspartame in order to reach the limits set by the FDA.

Other concerns surrounding the use of aspartame in the diet include those affecting a group of people who may lack the enzyme needed to metabolize the amino acid phenylalanine. This condition, called *PKU-phenylketonuria*, is genetic and rare, but it can be dangerous if this amino acid is consumed. (Babies are screened for this genetic abnormality at birth.) Because of this, labels are placed on all foods indicating that these products contain phenylalanine.

## Acesulfame K

In the late 1980s, another sugar substitute was introduced for use in dry and prepared foods, desserts, candies, soft drinks, chewing gum, and as a tabletop sweetener. This substitute, known as *Acesulfame K* (marketed as Sunette and Sweet One), is also 200 times sweeter than sugar, but because of an occasional aftertaste, it is often combined with other sweeteners. Acesulfame K provides no calories, is not metabolized by the body, and is excreted in the urine. This substitute also has been extensively studied for safety but has as of yet shown no toxic effects.

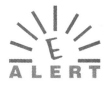

PKU-phenylketonuria is a rare genetic disease that does not allow certain people to metabolize the amino acid phenylalanine properly. People with this condition should avoid products containing NutraSweet (aspartame).

## Other Types of Artificial Sweeteners

Besides the possible reintroduction of cyclamate, other sweeteners are currently being considered for use in our country. These include sucralose and alitame.

Sucralose is actually a low-calorie sweetener made from sugar. It is about 600 times as sweet as sugar and contributes no calories. Highly stable during food processing, this sweetener makes a good choice for use in baked goods. Currently, sucralose can be found in over twenty-five countries outside the United States.

Alitame, a sweetener made from amino acids, offers a taste 2,000 times sweeter than sugar. This product can be useful in cooking, baking, in beverages, as a tabletop sweetener, and in frozen desserts.

## Using Sugar Substitutes

Although daily use of sugar substitutes has increased threefold in the last decade, studies have not indicated a significant change in body weight or decreased consumption of high-sugar products overall. It appears that many individuals opt for a combination of both—foods with sugar substitutes and those with regular table sugar.

For individuals seeking to lose weight, sugar substitutes can help, but only if they are used properly and as a substitute for table sugar. Sugar substitutes have a wide variety of uses, but consumers should understand that they do not function in the same manner as table sugar. Because of their composition, these substitutes cannot be substituted equally for sugar. For that reason, it is advised to do the following.

- Read the label of the sweetener package for sugar equivalents.
- Seek recipes developed by sweetener manufacturers and promoters for best outcome.
- Opt for more recipes that do not require heating, like frozen desserts, gelatins, beverages, smoothies, and salads.
- Experiment with foods and recipes you like. It may take several tries to get it right, but after a while you may find a new recipe you enjoy.

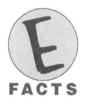

**FACTS**

No evidence has indicated that people who regularly use sugar substitutes over sugar actually lose more weight than those who do not.

As you can see, no single sugar substitute meets all the needs of consumers. Some are preferred as tabletop sweeteners, others for baked products, and still others for beverages and frozen foods. Although low-calorie sweeteners do have their place in the food supply, and even though they can help reduce the overall intake of sugar and reduce a person's "sweet tooth," individuals should keep in mind that these products are not the magic answer to weight control. Substituting with sweeteners alone cannot make up for a poor diet. Individuals seeking to lose weight still need to combine a balanced diet with an exercise program for best results.

## Removing the Fat from Food

Fat is a complicated nutrient to remove from our food. It is not only a necessary component to the diet, it adds taste, consistency, stability, and palatability to our foods. Fat is needed in the diet for proper growth and development, and it is important in maintaining overall good health. Additionally, we need fats to transport the fat-soluble vitamins (vitamins A, D, E, K) throughout the body and help in their absorption.

Even so, food manufacturers have felt the need to crack this market and offer comparative fat substitutes, often called *fat replacers*, into our food supply. It sounds like a good idea! Wouldn't it be great to offer the real benefit of fat without all those calories that contribute to excess weight gain?

Recent years have brought on an abundance of low-fat, reduced-fat, and nonfat products. All intentions were to help reduce the intake of fat (and maybe excess calories and weight) through use of these products. But our population has grown heavier over recent years, instead of thinner, which means the opposite has resulted. Why has this happened?

Let's learn more about these fat substitutes.

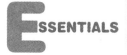

Beware of food containing fat substitutes. These foods may be lower in fat, but they are not necessarily lower in calories. Many of the calories are made up with sugar.

## Types of Fat Replacers

Just like sugar substitutes, several types of fat replacers have been introduced into the marketplace. Currently there are three different types: those that are carbohydrate based, those that are protein based, and those that are fat based. These fat substitutes are made to help reduce the overall fat content of a food while still providing the texture, taste, and feel of eating fat. But to date, none has proved to offer as much as fat itself.

**E**SSENTIALS

The fat contained in foods is key to providing taste and texture. Fat substitutes cannot always accomplish this, thus often providing food products that are less satisfying to consumers.

## Carbohydrate-Based Fat Substitutes

An early fat substitute (in the mid 1960s) was a carbohydrate-based product referred to as *Avicel*, a cellulose-gel used as a food stabilizer. Other products followed, like Carrageenan, a seaweed derivative, Litesse, and products like dextrins, gums, and starch. Carbohydrate-based substitutes are made from thickeners used to supply a bulky feel to the diet, similar to the feel of fat. Caloric values of these substitutes range from 0 to 4 calories per gram, as compared to 9 calories per gram from fat, thus reducing fat calories by more than half as long as comparable amounts are consumed. These substitutes are used in a variety of foods, including luncheon meats, salad dressings, frozen desserts, baked goods, and candies, but they are not suitable for use in frying.

## Protein-Based Fat Substitutes

Protein-based fat substitutes originated in the early 1990s and were designed solely to replace fats in foods. These products are made from egg whites or skim milk, and they supply up to half of the calories of regular fat. Familiar to many consumers under the trade name "Simplesse," products like these help provide a creamy feel to the food, particularly after the fat is removed. This kind of fat substitute is found in foods like butter, sour cream, cheeses, salad dressings, mayonnaise, baked goods, snack chips, frozen desserts, coffee creamers, and candies.

## Fat-Based Fat Substitutes

Olestra, also called *Olean*, the fat-based substitute, was thought to have been the best option so far, as its qualities are as yet the closest to naturally occurring fat, but controversies surrounding its use have kept it from being as popular as once hoped. Made primarily from sugar and vegetable oil, this fat substitute is made into molecules that are too large to be digested. No digestion results in no fat calories being absorbed. Food sources containing Olestra include salty snacks like potato chips, tortilla chips, cheese puffs, and snack crackers, along with cake mixes and dairy foods. Olestra can also be used in frying foods. Sounds good so far!

Since being released into the market, complaints surfaced regarding digestive problems, abdominal cramping, and intestinal discomfort. Also, concerns have been raised about Olestra's effect on reducing the absorption of the essential fat-soluble vitamins (vitamins A, D, E, K). Because of these concerns, studies will need to continue monitoring the safety of long-term consumption of Olestra-containing foods. In the meantime, food products must be labeled to indicate current safety concerns.

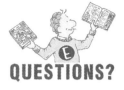

**QUESTIONS?**

**Why can't fat just be taken out of foods?**
Fat is necessary for taste and to maintain food texture. It is also an important component in providing texture during cooking, in that fat helps to make a food crispy and crunchy. By removing it altogether, the entire property of the food would be changed and its taste would be less than desirable.

Additional fat replacers have also found their place in the marketplace, and many more will likely show up in upcoming years. Consumer demand brings on the need for new options and new varieties. Currently many fat replacers are in the developmental stages, but as long as consumer interest remains high, these will likely find their way into our foods.

## Safety Concerns

Consumers continue to be concerned about the safety of sugar substitutes and fat replacers. The Food and Drug Administration (FDA) requires extensive studies on any new (and currently used) substitute. Products are studied based on their intended use and audience, and they are studied in areas relating to toxicity, safety issues, and problems associated with reproduction, metabolism, allergies, and cancer. In addition, the FDA examines how the product is made and how it will be processed and used. Through all this testing, determinations and guidelines are set regarding acceptable limits on the use of these products.

Keep in mind that consumers are responsible for their own consumption of products as well. Although a product may be promoted and advertised as safe, it is up to consumers to determine for themselves what products may or may not work. If adverse reactions are observed following use of a particular product, consumers should seek adequate care to determine the cause.

Foods containing sugar substitutes and fat replacers indeed can be beneficial to many consumers—if and only if they are used as a substitute and not as an addition to a diet containing high-sugar and high-fat foods, too. As part of an overall healthy eating plan, though, these substitutes can offer an effective means to reducing overall calories and fat in the diet.

**FACTS**

Fat substitutes can be beneficial if used properly. For example, substituting fat-free mayonnaise for regular mayonnaise, per tablespoon, can reduce calories from 100 to 10 calories and fat grams from 11 to 0 grams.

# Reducing Total Sugar and Fat Calories

It is possible to reduce total amounts of sugar and fats in the diet, if properly planned. But it isn't possible if your knowledge of good nutrition habits escape you as you select these products. Don't always assume that lower-sugar and lower-fat foods are lower in calories. In fact, many foods provide enough of the other calorie-producing nutrients, like other forms of sugar or sugar itself, to compensate for flavor, structure, and texture, which can often make little overall difference in the total caloric value. If honey or fructose is substituted for table sugar (sucrose), your calories will not change. If you buy a food product just because it says "light," don't always assume it is lighter in calories. Sometimes it is just lighter in color or texture. Compare nutrition labels to see the difference.

## Beware of Portions

Also, watch those portion sizes. Just because a product is lower in sugar or fat doesn't give you a green light to eat twice as much. Won't that defeat your purpose in the first place? If a food doesn't satisfy you, don't eat it just because it is lower in fat. It would make more sense to top your salad with 1 tablespoon of regular salad dressing and enjoy the taste and variety of vegetables in the salad rather than to use 2 tablespoons of low-fat dressing you didn't like and force yourself to eat the salad, or maybe not eat it at all.

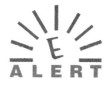

The Food and Drug Administration studies the safety of sugar and fat substitutes for people of all ages. Because children are growing and require a variety of nutrients, including fat, an abundance of substitutes should not be included in their diet. Moderate consumption of foods containing substitutes will not be harmful, but these foods should not replace a well-balanced collection of foods from all the essential food groups.

## Modify Your Diet

Here is a sample diet showing how you can incorporate healthy modifications without sacrificing your nutrient requirements:

| | REGULAR DIET | MODIFIED DIET |
|---|---|---|
| **BREAKFAST** | | |
| | ¾ cup orange juice | ¾ cup orange juice |
| | 1 bagel | 1 bagel |
| | 1 Tbsp. margarine | 1 Tbsp. reduced-fat margarine |
| | 1 Tbsp. jelly | 1 Tbsp. low-sugar spread |
| | coffee with 2 tsp. sugar | coffee with sugar substitute |
| | and 1 Tbsp. half-and-half | and nonfat creamer |
| **LUNCH** | | |
| | 2 slices whole-wheat bread | 2 slices whole-wheat bread |
| | 2 ounces sliced turkey | 2 ounces sliced turkey |
| | 1 ounce American cheese | 1 ounce reduced-fat cheese product |
| | 1 Tbsp. mayonnaise | 1 Tbsp. reduced-fat mayonnaise |
| | 1 ounce potato chips | 1 ounce baked potato chips |
| | apple | apple |
| | 12-ounce can regular soft drink | 12-ounce can diet soft drink |
| **SNACK** | | |
| | 3 sandwich cookies | 3 reduced-fat sandwich cookies |
| | 1 cup whole milk | 1 cup reduced-fat milk |

| | REGULAR DIET | MODIFIED DIET |
|---|---|---|
| **DINNER** | | |
| | 3 ounces grilled chicken | 3 ounces grilled chicken |
| | baked potato with | baked potato with 2 tsp. |
| | 2 tsp. sour cream | reduced-fat sour cream |
| | green salad with | green salad with 2 Tbsp. |
| | 1 Tbsp. salad dressing | reduced-fat salad dressing |
| | roll with 1 tsp. margarine | roll with 1 tsp. reduced-fat margarine |
| | 12-ounce can regular soft drink | 12-ounce can diet soft drink |
| **SNACK** | | |
| | ½ cup ice cream | ½ cup reduced-fat ice cream |
| **Total Calories:** | 2,449 | 1,797 |
| **Total Fat:** | 88 grams | 42 grams |

Because of the demand to decrease the amount of sugar and fat in our diets, sugar and fat substitutes are continually being researched and more will be introduced to the marketplace. Low-calorie sweeteners and fat replacers do have a place in your mission to control your overall calorie and fat consumption. But consumers need to understand what and how they should best be used. Just because a product uses a sugar or fat substitute does not necessarily make it a "diet food" or one that can be eaten in excessive amounts.

Many foods made with substitutes offer little or no nutrient content and little satiety value, and they often increase one's overall appetite. Many foods typically containing substitutes are those that had little nutritional value to begin with, like convenience foods, chips, baked goods, desserts, and beverages. These foods should not take the place of the healthier choices like lean sources of protein, whole grains, fruits, vegetables, and dairy products. An excessive consumption of these types of foods can result in eating larger quantities or eating more than otherwise would have been consumed. Consumers need to be aware of what they are eating and make wise choices that can fit into the entire diet.

## CHAPTER 11
# Going Vegetarian

he vegetarian lifestyle has been around for hundreds of years, but it is more popular today than ever before. Once considered an odd way of eating, today vegetarianism is known as a preferred eating and lifestyle approach for people of all ages. Food manufacturers and restaurants are even taking notice and offering meals and food products to meet the needs of these individuals.

## Why Become a Vegetarian?

Reasons to become a vegetarian are quite varied. Some people choose this lifestyle to avoid "eating animals." They feel it is not humane, or do so for religious reasons. Others believe in saving the environment, and still others find it to be a healthier way of life. Food guidelines that encourage people to consume high-fiber, low-fat diets that include many sources of whole grains, fruits, and vegetables and less fat from meat and dairy products can also push individuals into this eating approach.

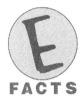

FACTS

An estimated 14 million Americans currently consider themselves as following a vegetarian lifestyle, with another million joining these food patterns each year.

Why go vegetarian? Some give reasons like the following:

- For environmental reasons
- To save animals
- For health reasons
- For religious or spiritual reasons
- For overall health

## The Health Benefits

Research does show a connection between vegetarianism and health. Risk of diseases like heart disease, hypertension (high blood pressure), diabetes, obesity, and some types of cancers are reduced, as well as problems associated with kidney stones and gallstones. Food choices for these people could contribute to these declines, but other factors, including genetics, physical activity, and not smoking, all have an impact as well.

People who choose to follow a vegetarian lifestyle are known to have the following benefits.

- A lower incidence of chronic disease.
- Less total fat and saturated fat in the diet.
- Receive greater benefits from plant-based foods (antioxidants and phytonutrients).
- Lower cholesterol levels.
- Lower incidence of high blood pressure.
- Reduced incidence of various types of cancers including lung, colon, and breast.
- Fewer incidence and complications from type II diabetes.

But just choosing to be a vegetarian and going vegetarian don't guarantee a healthy life and reduced risk of disease. This type of diet, along with a good sense of nutrition knowledge, is important. Proper planning of meals and snacks is just as important as it is with other dietary patterns, regardless of the type of diet you choose.

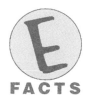

**FACTS**

With the exception of those who follow vegan vegetarian diets, most vegetarians have no difficulties obtaining adequate protein in their diets.

# A Vegetarian Food Pyramid

The Food Guide Pyramid again comes into play here. Moderate changes can be made to the general food pyramid to make it a helpful reference for vegetarians, too. The grain, fruit, and vegetable groups within the pyramid remain the same as the general Food Guide Pyramid, whereas several modifications are made to the protein and dairy groups to allow for nonmeat sources to be included. (The Vegetarian Food Guide Pyramid is illustrated using the Lacto-ovo-vegetarian food style. This type of vegetarian diet includes eggs and dairy products. Vegetarians following stricter dietary patterns should modify their intake accordingly.) Overall recommended serving and portion sizes from each group remain the same, as does the importance of seeking balance, variety, and moderation.

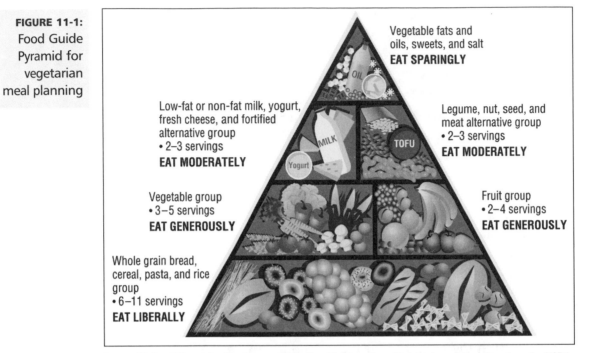

**FIGURE 11-1:**
Food Guide
Pyramid for
vegetarian
meal planning

Source: National Center for Nutrition and Dietetics, The American Dietetic Association. Based on the USDA Food Guide Pyramid

But can vegetarian diets really supply your body with the variety and amount of nutrients you need on a daily basis? Yes, they can, but again careful planning must take place. And of course it depends on how strict your vegetarian diet may be. There are several common types of vegetarianism. Some may be more challenging to follow than others.

**E**SSENTIALS Supplements can help meet nutrient needs of vegetarians, but they cannot replace the importance of receiving nutrition from the foods you eat.

## What Does Going Vegetarian Mean?

Vegetarianism means avoiding eating meat, poultry, fish, and products made from these animal sources, like milk, cheese, yogurt, and eggs. Some vegetarians strictly follow this pattern; others modify it to their specific preference. Some include fish, others include dairy products, and still others allow eggs.

## Types of Vegetarians Diets

There are clearly defined types of vegetarian diets, each identified by specific names, although many variations can exist with individuals following them. Here is a rundown of the most common types of vegetarian diets.

- **Lacto-ovo-vegetarian:** These individuals choose a diet that includes eggs and dairy products but that does not allow meat, poultry, or fish. This is the most common form of vegetarianism and is the one illustrated in the preceding Vegetarian Food Guide Pyramid.
- **Lacto-vegetarian:** These individuals avoid meat, poultry, fish, and eggs, but do include dairy products into their diets.
- **Vegans, or strict vegetarians:** The vegan approach to vegetarianism is the strictest form of vegetarianism in that individuals eat no animal products whatsoever: no meat, poultry, fish, eggs, or dairy products. Some also choose to avoid butter, margarine (made with whey products), and honey (as it is made by bees).
- **Semi-vegetarians or partial vegetarians:** Although not a specific type of vegetarianism, many people choose this approach to eating, as they choose to vary nonmeat meals with an occasional meal that includes meat, poultry, or fish.

You can make a complementary protein by combining two or more incomplete proteins that in turn provide all the essential amino acids that the body needs. Different foods supply different amino acids. Be smart in which you choose to eat together, and you can end up with a complete protein source.

## Incorporating Vegetarianism into Daily Meals

Whether you choose any of these options or not, there are many ways to incorporate vegetarian meals into your daily lifestyle. These meals can be lower in fat, higher in fiber, and very filling and satisfying. Because of the benefits in choosing lower-fat and higher-fiber foods, vegetarians can easily plan weight-reduction diets that are healthy, satisfying, and nutritious.

Let's focus in on each group of the food pyramid to identify some good choices to incorporate into your diet plans.

- **GRAIN GROUP** Whole-grain breads and cereals; enriched and fortified products; pasta; brown rice, white rice; barley, rice pilaf, pasta dishes, tabouli, couscous; tortillas, pitas, bagels, English muffins, challah, focaccia; yeast bread, raisin bread, cornbread; popcorn, pretzels; wheat germ, wheat bran.
- **FRUIT GROUP** Melons, watermelons, honeydew, cantaloupe; berries, strawberries, blueberries, blackberries, raspberries; citrus fruits, oranges, grapefruits; kiwi; dried fruits, raisins, apricots, prunes, plums; fruits as toppings for cakes, ice creams, and in smoothies.
- **VEGETABLE GROUP** Green leafy vegetables, kale, collards, mustard, turnip greens, spinach, bok choy, broccoli; carrots, celery, onions; tomatoes; peppers (green, red, yellow); zucchini; fresh, canned, frozen vegetables.
- **PROTEIN GROUP** Soy products, tofu, tempeh, textured soy protein; vegetarian meal alternatives, veggie burgers; peanut butters, nut spreads; eggs, egg whites, egg substitutes; legumes, dried beans, peas, garbanzo, pinto, black, white, split, vegetarian refried beans, bean soups; nuts, almonds, walnuts, peanuts, pecans, cashews; seeds, sunflower, pumpkin, sesame.
- **DAIRY GROUP** Soy-based milk, yogurt, cheese; rice milk.

## The Challenges of Vegetarian Eating

We've discussed the benefits and advantages to choosing a vegetarian lifestyle as well as types and various foods that can be found in this type of diet. But we have yet to touch on the many challenges that can accompany those following a vegetarian diet. The type of vegetarian lifestyle you choose will determine what type of challenges you will encounter. If your diet tends to be strict and more in line with the vegan lifestyle, it may be more difficult for you to meet all your nutritional needs given that a lack of animal foods in the diet also leads to a lack of vitamin $B_{12}$. Other nutrients of concern include vitamin D, calcium, iron, and zinc. Individuals who are semi-vegetarians or who include eggs and dairy products in their meals may have less difficulty. Whatever plan you follow, you must be cautious about your intake of fats, just like in other diets. And sugar and sodium should also be consumed in moderation. In any case, when carefully planned, each and every type of vegetarian diet can contribute to a healthy intake and lifestyle.

**E**SSENTIALS    High-quality complete proteins are necessary in the diet for normal growth and development.

## Protein

Because animal sources are our primary source of protein, and because they are the ones that include high-quality complete protein, careful attention needs to be paid in order for this important nutrient to be a part of vegetarian diet plans. Lacto-ovo and lacto-vegetarians who consume dairy products and eggs have fewer difficulties consuming adequate amounts of protein than vegan vegetarians. But even so, with proper planning, vegans can meet their protein needs without great difficulty.

Plants can contribute protein to the diet, but they are not a complete protein. Beans and legumes like kidney beans, navy beans, chickpeas, lentils, soybeans, nuts, and seeds are also considered good protein sources, but again they are not complete sources. A complete protein is one in which all the essential amino acids are found within the protein. An incomplete source does not contain all of the essential amino acids, meaning one of two could be missing.

Your body needs the right combination all amino acids (the nine essentials, supplied by food sources, and eleven nonessentials, made by the body) in order to build tissues and other compounds. If one or more is missing, your cells will not be able to make a complete protein. But this is not cause for alarm. Through a process of combining various incomplete sources of protein with each other, your body can make a complete protein source. In other words, by combining one food that offers some of the essential amino acids with another food that offers the other essential amino acids, you can create a complete protein source. Some of these combinations include the following:

- Dried beans and barley
- Dried peas and oats
- Lentils and corn
- Peanuts and rice
- Soy/soy products and pasta
- Soy/soy products and whole-grain/enriched breads
- Soy/soy products and nuts (almonds, walnuts, pecans, cashews) or seeds (sesame, sunflower)

A general rule of thumb is to combine legumes with grains, nuts, or seeds. Here are some examples:

- Peanut butter on whole wheat bread
- Black bean or split pea soup with sesame seed crackers
- Red beans with rice

**ESSENTIALS**

Vegetarians can make complete proteins in their diet by combining legumes with grains, nuts, or seeds.

When combining complementary proteins, it is not always necessary to consume these foods together at the same meal or at the same time. But it is important to consume various selections from the legumes with selections from the grain group over the course of a meal or two in order to reap the benefits of creating a complete protein.

## Calcium, Iron, and Zinc

Calcium, iron, and zinc are important nutrients that are also primarily found in animal foods. In the event that dairy foods and eggs are not eaten, careful attention must be made to ensure that foods supplying these nutrients are included in the diet.

Calcium is necessary for developing and maintaining strong bones and teeth, along with regulating the heartbeat and helping with muscle contractions. Iron is necessary for carrying oxygen throughout the body, and zinc is important in controlling various body processes, including assisting with body growth and sexual development and aiding in enzyme activities.

Lacto-ovo- and lacto-vegetarians can easily meet their calcium needs through dairy products. But for those vegetarians who do not consume dairy products, dark green leafy vegetables like broccoli, bok choy, kale, and collard and mustard greens can supply calcium. Tofu and soy milk are also good sources. In addition, many foods are supplemented with calcium today, including orange juice and cereals.

Iron and zinc are primarily supplied in animal products like meat. For vegetarians, these minerals can easily be added to the diet through a wide selection of fortified breakfast cereals (read the labels), dried beans, dried fruits, and prune juice.

## Vitamins D and $B_{12}$

Vitamin D and vitamin $B_{12}$ are also two vitamins that can easily be lacking in vegetarian diets. Vitamin D is important in calcium absorption and for bone health. Vitamin $B_{12}$ is important in growth, maintaining nerve tissue, and keeping blood healthy. A deficiency of vitamin D can result in poor bone growth, whereas lack of vitamin $B_{12}$ can lead to anemia and, over the long term, possibly to nerve damage.

Vitamin D can be obtained, though, by exposure to the sun. When the sun shines on the skin, a provitamin is formed in the skin that the liver and kidneys then make into vitamin D. For those who do not spend a great deal of time in the sun, this vitamin can be obtained from fortified soy milk and from fortified cereals. Vitamin $B_{12}$ can also be found in fortified soy milk and cereals.

Vegan vegetarians in particular can be deficient in vitamin $B_{12}$, vitamin D, calcium, iron, and zinc. Care must be taken to obtain these nutrients in this type of diet.

In some cases, for strict vegetarians and those with concerns about their diet and low intake of certain vitamins and minerals, a vitamin-mineral supplement may be warranted. If you choose to seek a dietary supplement to help meet your particular nutrient needs, seek a product that contains no more than 100 percent of the Recommended Dietary Allowance (RDA). Remember supplements can help meet nutrient needs, but they are no substitute for a healthy, well-balanced intake of foods.

## Fat

As I indicated before, many people assume that going vegetarian means following a healthier lifestyle, maybe even one that can help with weight loss. Not necessarily so. Fat can be a problem for vegetarians just as it can be a problem for nonvegetarians. Many vegetarians opt for sources of protein like cheese, soy products, nuts, and seeds, but they do so without noticing the amount of fat some of these products contain.

Recommendations regarding fat remain the same for vegetarians and nonvegetarians alike. Keeping fat intake to less than 30 percent of total calories is suggested, along with including low-fat choices of dairy products, including milk, cheese, cottage cheese, and yogurt. Also, keep a watchful eye on extras like margarine, oils, cream, sour cream, and sauces that may be added to foods. These extras can add more fat than you might realize.

## Vegetarian Meal Planning

Yes, I've said it's important to plan meals and snacks if you are a vegetarian, but it is important for nonvegetarians to plan meals and snacks, too. Planning meals and snacks for several days or a week at a time allows you to properly shop, stock staples, and plan your time more effectively. If you need some help initially, I've included a sample meal plan and some snack options to help guide you.

## Meal Ideas

A sample **LACTO-OVO** and **LACTO-VEGETARIAN** diet may be as follows:

- **Breakfast:** ¾ cup orange juice; 1 ounce fortified cereal; 1 cup low-fat milk.
- **Lunch:** Veggie wrap (tortilla with shredded lettuce, zucchini, tomatoes, chickpeas, and 1 tablespoon of reduced-fat salad dressing) and ¾ cup fresh strawberries.
- **Snack:** 8 ounces vanilla yogurt with 1 tablespoon granola topping and a banana.
- **Dinner:** 1 cup black bean soup, stir-fry vegetables and tofu over pasta, and a dinner roll with margarine.
- **Snack:** Bagel with hummus spread and 1 cup low-fat milk.

A sample **VEGAN DIET** may be as follows:

- **Breakfast:** ¾ cup orange juice, 1 ounce fortified cereal, 1 cup fortified soy milk.
- **Lunch:** Veggie wrap (tortilla with shredded lettuce, zucchini, tomatoes, chickpeas, and 1 tablespoon reduced-fat salad dressing) and ¾ cup fresh strawberries.
- **Snack:** ½ cup trail mix (nuts, fortified cereal, dried fruits) and a banana.
- **Dinner:** 1 cup black bean soup, stir-fry vegetables and tofu over pasta, and a dinner roll with margarine (optional).
- **Snack:** Bagel with hummus spread and 1 cup fortified soy milk.

This menu offers approximately 2,200 calories and 65 grams of fat. Although it is a healthy meal plan, it would need to be modified slightly for weight reduction. This can easily be accomplished through reduction of starches (eliminate granola topping on yogurt, substitute raisins only for trail mix, eliminate dinner roll or substitute it for the pasta, decrease bagel at snack time to half rather than a whole bagel).

## Snack Ideas

High-quality snacks are a must for planning a healthy vegetarian diet, as they are with any type of diet. Choosing snack foods that contribute to the overall nutrition status of an individual is key to maintaining and reducing weight. Quantity and size of portions must also be considered when choosing snacks, just as they are with meals. Here is a collection of healthy choices that not only are delicious and nutritious but that are also high in fiber and lower in fat.

- Smoothie made with frozen fruit, juice, soy milk
- Salad with a fruit topping, like strawberries or mandarin oranges
- Salad with bean topping, like chickpeas
- Fortified dry cereal
- Veggie pizza bagel or English muffin
- Cup of bean, pasta, vegetable soup
- Vegetable sticks and low-fat dip/hummus
- Crackers and soy cheese
- Peanut or soy butter on celery sticks or graham crackers
- Quick-breads made with fruit, shredded zucchini, or carrots

As you can see, maintaining a vegetarian lifestyle requires careful planning and direction. For individuals who choose to follow this style of eating, careful attention needs to be paid to obtain the wide variety of essential nutrients. Choosing foods on a daily basis from the Vegetarian Food Guide Pyramid helps to accomplish this. Portions also need to be moderate in size. (Refer to Chapter 6 for direction on selecting adequate portion sizes.) Vegetarian resources and recipes are abundant and can be found at local libraries, bookstores, and on the Internet. Should you desire to pursue this lifestyle approach, I would highly recommend further educating yourself in this area.

CHAPTER 12

# Problems Associated with Eating Disorders

**P**eople have been suffering from eating disorders for many years. But only over the last several decades have these disorders become better understood and treated.

# What Causes an Eating Disorder?

The increased incidence of eating disorders has been blamed on various factors. Some relate to emotions and feelings, others to a strong desire to be thin, others to never-ending dieting patterns, and still others to unrealistic expectations placed on individuals, particularly teenagers. No single factor has been shown to be the cause of these disorders, but each can contribute in its own way. In fact, the causes seem to be varied for different people.

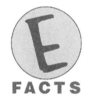

**FACTS**

Although the majority of victims are females, some 90 percent, the incidence of eating disorders in males is beginning to rise. Younger people are also falling victim, with teenagers accounting for the largest number of cases, at somewhere around 85 percent. Reactions to feeling rejected, worthless, and unhappy about appearance can result in out-of-control behaviors such as using excessive food for comfort or overly controlling intake of food.

## Behaviors/Emotions/Feelings

Each person has his or her own type of eating and behavior patterns. Many are highly affected by feelings and emotions. Strong emotions often cause some people to eat in excess, while others resort to not eating at all. But this does not indicate that these individuals will suffer from an eating disorder.

## Peer/Competitive Pressure

Much of the increased blame of eating disorders is placed on society's strong desire to be thin. Models, actors, and rock stars form society's impression of attractiveness and success, while larger-sized individuals are often shown to be dull, boring, and undesirable. Many people begin to value a person's self-worth on their body size and shape. This strong impact causes many people who may be within normal weight to diet beyond healthy limits. When one diet doesn't work, another is tried, and this process continues over and over again until disordered eating patterns result.

Body image is defined as one's internal view of his or her body size, shape, and weight. Those with negative body images perceive their bodies as it is not—too big, too fat, unattractive, or a reflection of personal failure. And those with positive body images see their bodies as they are—accepting of its size, shape, weight, not perfect but a body they feel comfortable in.

Competitive athletes are also highly prone to eating disorders in that their standards far exceed those of amateurs. Constant demands to achieve weight goals for their particular sport or competition, especially among groups like dancers and gymnasts, can be enough reason for self-starvation at some times and at other times to binge and purge.

## Common Theories

Some theories indicate that a connection may exist between one's genetic background and his or her risk of developing an eating disorder. Certain chemicals in the brain may trigger overeating patterns. Still other theories concern families and the high expectations placed on children. When parents overly stress the importance of high achievement and appearance, children often find alternate avenues in which they can control their lives. Eating disorders are known to result from these pressures.

While many people move in and out of abnormal eating patterns throughout their lives, only one in ten form actual eating disorders.

People must realize that eating disorders are not only a nutrition problem but a psychological one as well. Yes, these teens (and adults) want to be thin, and almost nothing can stand in their way of accomplishing their goals to strive to be their thinnest. But just going on a reducing diet is not necessarily enough to cause an eating disorder. These disorders are often much more complex than that.

## Who Does It Affect?

Eating disorders affect not only the individuals themselves. They also weigh heavily on the entire family. When a person suffers from an eating disorder, his or her entire world becomes involved. Work life, family life, relationships, health, emotional states, and more are highly affected.

Often, an eating disorder results from a life-changing experience or trauma, such as a death in the family, divorce, or moving away to college, but that is not the only reason. Striving for perfection or placing stress on an individual to perform beyond his or her abilities can also contribute to problems. When this happens, the person feels like he cannot control his inner feelings and emotions. Food then serves as a comfort or control mechanism, whether that means eating more or eating less. Eating disorders are classified as psychiatric disorders, but they also include large nutritional and medical components.

**ESSENTIALS**

Eating disorders are not just about being thin and trim. They include issues relating to self-esteem, depression, power, and control, as well.

## Who Is at Risk?

Anyone is at risk for eating disorders. These problems do not just affect females, teens, and those seeking to diet. Yes, indeed, these disorders occur more frequently within these groups, with females accounting for the largest number at somewhere around 90 to 95 percent, but other groups of individuals can also be affected.

Teens are highly influenced by television and celebrity models. They want to be thin as they can be, they strive for perfection within themselves, and they also have many outside pressures from school, parents, and peers. Athletes, particularly dancers and gymnasts, many of whom are also teens, are at risk as well, as these individuals constantly seek options to keep low body weights.

Teenagers are prone to problems associated with eating disorders in that they are very vulnerable and impressionable.

And young males should not be forgotten. This group is at risk in similar ways in that they also seek perfectionism and can be involved in competitive sports, like wrestling (where it's important to keep weight down). In addition, these young men may be seeking an outlet to control emotions. Men and boys are raised to keep feelings and emotions buried, rarely crying in public or sharing feelings of sadness, guilt, or pain. Often, this hiding of emotions can play out in control of eating compulsively or not eating at all.

## Do You Think You May Be at Risk?

Determining whether you may be at risk is a complicated process. Obsession with weight, body size, calorie counting, exercising, and eating can all be related to risk. Ask yourself the following questions. The more questions you answer with a "yes" response, the greater your risk for developing an eating disorder:

- Do I often compare my shape and size to other people and strive to be thinner than everyone I associate with?
- Do I feel "fat" even after people tell me I am not?
- Do I frequently go on restrictive diets?
- Do I constantly think about food?
- Do I have irregular or no menstrual cycles?
- Do I insist on exercising daily and for lengthy periods of time?
- Do I pick at my food and take tiny bites or not eat any food on my plate at all?
- Do I avoid going places to prevent confrontation with food?
- Do I hide food or eat often when alone and in excessive amounts?
- Do I weigh myself more than once each day?
- Does the number on the scale influence my attitude for that day?
- Do I tell people I have eaten a meal, even if I have not?

- Do I feel guilty if I overeat?
- Do I take laxatives?
- Do I make myself purge (vomit after eating) to avoid feeling guilty about what I have eaten?

Answering yes to these questions should raise a red flag of caution for an eating disorder problem. If you feel you may need some help, there are many resources available. In the event that you notice many of these behaviors in another person close to you, you may want to seek support or treatment options here too. Information for support is available from your physician, a registered dietitian, or through the resources listed in Appendix B.

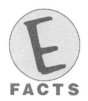

**FACTS**

Current estimates show that over five million Americans suffer from eating disorders, including anorexia nervosa, bulimia nervosa, and binge eating disorders.

## Early Signs of Eating Disorders

Signs of an eating disorder can be visible or hidden. Depending on the type and severity of the disorder, the signs may or may not be clear enough to determine the problem. Some individuals may lose significant amounts of weight, others may remain at normal weight, and others may gain weight.

There are some early signs, though, that may signal a problem. These include the following:

- Changes in eating behaviors
- Drastic changes in body weight
- Frequent attempts at restrictive dieting
- Loss of appetite or denial of hunger
- Frequent weighing
- Wearing baggy clothes to hide overly thin body
- Overexercising

- Frequent visits to the washroom, especially after eating
- Use of laxatives or diuretics
- Constipation
- Dry skin, rashes, dry hair, thinning hair
- Depressed behavior, withdrawal from friends

Eating disorders can be classified into three distinct types, although variations and combinations of each can occur. These include anorexia nervosa, bulimia nervosa, and binge eating disorder.

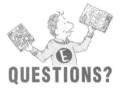

**QUESTIONS?**

**What are some common behaviors associated with eating disorders?**
Common behaviors prevalent in those suffering from eating disorders include unsafe and very restrictive dieting practices, use of unsafe or unproven diet medications or products, and attempts to seek an unrealistic body size or shape.

# Anorexia Nervosa: The Starvation Disorder

Anorexia Nervosa (anorexia) is also often referred to as *self-starvation*. This particular eating disorder is surrounded by the fear of gaining weight, with the victims feeling "fat" when in fact they are of very normal size or even very underweight. Distorted images of themselves are common. Obsessive behaviors of eating and intense exercise activity can consume these individuals.

## Signs and Symptoms

Anorexics are noted for having psychological problems as well, both social and emotional. As a result, they often withdraw from their families and friends and use the disorder as a means to gain power and control over their problems.

Initially anorexics may restrict their diet just to lose a few pounds. As the pounds fall away, they begin to feel more control over and pride in their accomplishments. Compliments regarding their weight inspire them to seek further success and achievements. This pattern continues until it gets out of hand, and feelings of pride turn into an obsession. Victims of anorexia rarely realize the implications of the disorder, and denial is frequent.

Although each individual varies in his or her particular signs and symptoms, it is common to see anorexics skip meals, pick at their food, eat very little, hide food, and indicate they have eaten a meal when in fact they have not. Others opt for laxatives or diuretics to help the dieting process along. Exercise increases to the point of excess, including activities like jogging, swimming, or aerobic conditioning.

As the disorder continues, physical symptoms become more visible. Low body weight is obvious and often victims wear baggy clothes to hide their frail bodies. A low amount of body fat can result in a condition called *amenorrhea*, or the ceasing of menstrual periods. Stress, restlessness, and irritability are common. Anorexics often complain of cold body temperatures, likely due to loss of body fat, particularly from the layer of fat under the skin that helps insulate the body. Dry skin, rashes, dry hair, and loss of hair are also noted.

**E**SSENTIALS

Eating disorders are defined as abnormal eating behaviors that cause physical and mental health problems. They are destructive patterns with complex causes.

In the case of a teenager with anorexia, growth and development patterns may be affected. Blood pressure rates drop, muscle masses can deteriorate, and bone density decreases. Body organs can also be impacted. Unless appropriate treatment is given, ongoing anorexia can wreak havoc on the body and mind and can result in death due to suicide or even starvation.

## Common Signs of Anorexia

Common signs of anorexia include the following:

- Rapid loss of weight to 85 percent or less of acceptable body weight.

- Wearing loose-fitting clothes to disguise weight loss.
- Eating very small amounts at a time.
- Often refusing to eat.
- Specific rituals involving food, eating, and exercise.
- Perfectionism.
- Lying about having eaten a meal.
- Rare recognition or acknowledgement of signs of hunger.
- Intense fear of being fat or gaining weight.
- Frequent weighing, sometimes multiple times each day.
- Distorted body image.
- Preoccupation with food.
- Frequent preparation and handling of food for other people, but rarely for self.
- Refusal to admit to abnormal eating patterns.
- Obsessive exercising.
- Frequent constipation.
- Possible amenorrhea, lack of menstrual periods or irregular periods.
- Depression/withdrawn from others.
- Sensitivity to cold temperatures.
- Dry skin, rashes.
- Dry hair, hair loss.

# Bulimia: The Bingeing-Purging Disorder

Bulimia Nervosa (bulimia) is noted for two common behaviors. Bingeing, or uncontrollable eating patterns, is followed by purging, or removing the food intake from the intestinal tract to avoid weight gain. Purging can be accomplished by self-induced vomiting or through use of excessive laxatives, diuretics, or enemas to eliminate the food from the body. Some bulimics also follow patterns of intensive exercise to burn off the excess caloric intake. It is not uncommon to see a combination of bulimic behaviors with those already identified in anorexics.

## Signs and Symptoms

Once a person begins the pattern of bingeing and purging, it is often difficult to stop. This pattern can become a habit, and it is easier to accomplish as time goes on. Like anorexics, bulimics constantly center their lives around food. But with bulimics, food is consumed in massive quantities, up to thousands of calories in a few hours alone. These foods are often high in fat and calories, frequently classified as empty-calorie foods. It is not uncommon for a victim to consume an entire cake, package of cookies, and a dozen doughnuts or more in one sitting alone. Behavior patterns surrounding eating become totally out of control. Because many victims realize their patterns are not normal, they hide it from others. They eat in private and remove themselves to the washroom to purge. Their body weight usually remains constant so family members and friends do not as easily recognize it as a warning sign.

Serious health problems can result from long-term bulimic behaviors. Repeated episodes of vomiting can damage the throat and the esophagus and destroy tooth enamel. Water and electrolyte balance is also disrupted. Over time, various organs in the body, like the heart and liver, can become affected. If left untreated, long-term bulimia can even lead to death.

## Common Signs of Bulimia

Common signs of bulimia include the following:

- Appearance of normal or average weight
- Eating large amounts of food in one sitting, usually alone
- Disappearing after eating, often to the washroom
- Preoccupation with food, weight, and appearance
- Feeling out of control when eating
- Possible amenorrhea or irregular menstrual periods
- Hand lesions that result from putting hand down throat to induce vomiting
- Frequent use of laxatives, diuretics, enemas, vomit-inducing syrups
- Complaints of stomach and digestive problems, bloating, constipation, and diarrhea

- Understanding that eating patterns are abnormal
- Depression/withdrawal from others
- Frequent mood swings
- Low self-esteem
- Frequent headaches
- Dental problems associated with decaying tooth enamel

# Binge Eating Disorder: Compulsive Overeating

Another common eating disorder is referred to as *binge eating disorder*. This type of disorder involves consuming very large amounts of food, almost compulsively, but without any associated behaviors to avoid the weight gain. Here, individuals eat until they can eat no more and until they are uncomfortably full. Their eating behaviors become out of their control.

## Signs and Symptoms

Binge eaters do feel guilty about their consumption of food. They feel rejected, depressed, and shamed, and they become easily frustrated with themselves. Often, these individuals try to follow weight-loss diets but with little overall success. When failures do occur, compulsive eating begins again and patterns continue.

## Common Signs of Binge Eating Disorder

Commons sings of binge eating disorder include the following:

- Frequent overeating, especially when alone
- Gaining large amounts of weight, possibly becoming obese
- Eating until uncomfortably full
- Often eating when not hungry
- Feeling out of control when eating
- Preoccupation with foods, dieting, eating, and body weight
- Understanding that eating patterns are abnormal
- Frequently following restrictive diets without much success
- Feeling guilty after overeating

- Stomach and digestive problems
- Ongoing feelings of depression, frustration, rejection, guilt
- Low self-esteem

## Seeking Proper Treatment

People who suffer from eating disorders do need professional help. Without proper care, long-term negative consequences and even death can occur. But treatment does vary from individual to individual, depending on the severity and type of eating disorder. However, it is important to seek a reputable source of treatment and opt for a team approach, including a physician, registered dietitian, and psychologist who specialize in this area.

The physician will assist with problems associated with physical health. She will monitor weight, blood pressure, and other vital signs in addition to evaluating physical damage and prescribing medications, if necessary. The dietitian can offer support in creating and developing healthy food habits and patterns. Patients will explore their concerns about their bodies, weight issues, and food and learn what a healthy weight and healthy eating habits can be. The psychologist begins to tackle emotional issues that may have been the root of the problem. Also involved could be an exercise physiologist to help in developing an appropriate exercise program and possibly even a dentist to assist with dental issues that may have developed.

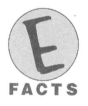

**FACTS**

Over half of all the individuals treated for eating disorders are able to recover, and they live and maintain a healthy life. But most individuals who are treated find that recovery is a lifelong process. The earlier treatment starts, the more successful it can be. Family support is also key in providing the best care available. Family support helps individual patients stick to their treatment over the long haul.

Hospitalization is often necessary, especially for anorexics, as these individuals may need to be fed intravenously or by another method if the patient refuses to eat. Anorexics often require medications that can stimulate the appetite. Nutrition and individual, group, and family psychological counseling are also integral components of treatment. Bulimics usually do not need hospitalization, but they do require nutrition and psychological counseling. Medications like antidepressants are often used with these individuals to help altered mood states and depression.

Unlike many illnesses, recovery is neither quick nor simple. Each person's recovery depends on many factors, including family and individual compliance, and on the severity of the disorder. The path to recovery is rocky. It takes a great deal of effort and understanding from everyone involved.

## Goals of Successful Treatment

In order to return those with eating disorders to a "normal" life and to "normal" eating behaviors, there are several goals that professionals seek to accomplish, including teaching patients the following:

- To lead a healthy and successful life
- To have healthy relationships with others
- To eat normally again
- The value of exercise within limits
- To become less obsessed with their body size
- To stop being concerned about how they compare to others
- To learn to eat all types of foods in moderation
- To learn to teach others the value and importance of healthy eating and healthy weight

Admitting a problem with an eating disorder is very difficult, but it becomes the first step in getting adequate help. Seeking out professional help is key in tackling the eating disorder along with whatever may have initially led to it.

If you know of a person with signs of an eating disorder, your best attempt at helping her or him is to offer support without being judgmental, critical, or pushy. Being a good listener is important. Remember that you are not the therapist—don't try to take over this role. Confront your friend, assist her or him in finding appropriate treatment, and be supportive throughout the recovery period.

CHAPTER 13

# *Handling an Overweight Child*

P roblems associated with body weight are increasing at an alarming rate, especially with our younger population. Children and teens have never been heavier. One in four American children is now considered overweight and at risk for future health problems.

## Potential Causes of Weight Gain

Many people may jump to the conclusion that their child's problems with obesity are genetic. It is true that in some people some causes of weight gain are genetic, but primary causes tend to be associated with our environment, including lifestyle habits, sedentary activity levels, frequency of eating out, and a high abundance of convenience and empty-calorie foods. Busier lifestyles are also to blame. Many households consist of working parents, with no one taking primary responsiblity for regular grocery shopping, meal planning, and food preparation.

Convenience-type foods, take-out orders, fast foods, and quick meals have taken over at mealtime. A decline of home-cooked dinners has also been observed. In all cases these trends are leading our younger generation to a higher consumption of fat and a decreased intake of lean meats, lower-fat dairy foods, and complex carbohydrates, including whole grains, fruits, and vegetables.

**E**SSENTIALS

Poor eating habits and low levels of physical activity are the primary causes of excessive weight gain in children today.

We also know that children are spending more and more time in front of the computer, surfing the Internet, watching television and cable programs, and testing the latest video games. These indoor (and sedentary) activities are taking our children away from outdoor play, bike riding, and other sports and physically active programs.

## How to Recognize a Problem

An obese child can be noticed at first glance. An overweight child may not as easily be recognized because a few extra pounds may just be temporary. This overweight child may just be moving through the bodily changes associated with puberty, or he could be on his way to a lifetime of problems associated with weight. It's important to take notice of weight patterns over the childhood years to keep on top of any problems that may occur.

**FACTS**

Preteen and teen bodies are supposed to grow and develop, thus increasing in height and weight too. Weight patterns may fluctuate, but may only be temporary. This is normal.

## Common Growth Concerns

As children grow, they change. Some kids grow taller, then fill out; others fill out first, then grow taller. In any case, the fact that a child is tall and thin or plump does not necessarily mean this child will be built like this as an adult. It is perfectly normal for a child's height and weight to constantly fluctuate as she grows, especially during the early teen years. If a child gains a few extra pounds at age twelve or thirteen, this may not be cause for alarm. But if a child puts on an extra 3 to 5 pounds a year for several years, this pattern may need to be broken before it gets out of hand.

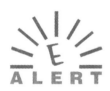

**ALERT**

The U.S. Surgeon General has officially declared childhood obesity as an epidemic and as a public health threat. Risks include type II diabetes, premature heart disease, bone and joint injuries, and psychological disorders. Children are also at increased risk of having physical limitations due to extra body weight and are more prone to depression and lower self-esteem.

## Assessing a Problem

If you are concerned that your child may be overweight or at risk for developing a weight problem, speak to your child's doctor. A doctor will be able to assess your child's growth patterns over the years to determine future risk for weight concerns. But again, height/weight charts are just one assessment that can be used. These growth patterns need to continue over several years in order to adequately determine risk.

Growth charts for children up to eighteen years of age (designed by the National Center for Health Statistics in collaboration with the Centers for Disease Control and Prevention) are available from pediatricians and physicians. These charts were designed to compare children to other children of the exact same age. Because of the variations between children at various ages, these charts illustrate that about half of all children will fall above and half below the fiftieth percentile for height and weight at each particular age. The fiftieth percentile would be considered average for that age. Taller children tend to lean toward higher percentages, shorter children toward lower percentages. But weight should follow suit. A child's weight should be somewhat consistent to her height. This is illustrated in the height versus weight comparison.

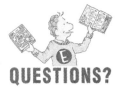

**QUESTIONS?**

**How can I determine if my child is actually overweight for his/her size?**
You can use a standard height/weight/BMI chart over the course of many years to determine growth patterns. Children who plot into a growth chart at the ninetieth percentile or greater on weight for height may be at risk for becoming overweight.

## Managing a Problem

Parents also need to look at family weight history. If other family members, particularly parents, are overweight, the risk for a child becoming overweight may also be greater. Now may be the time to incorporate some lifestyle changes for the benefit of the entire family. In the case of a child who has not yet entered into puberty, your best attempt is to focus on healthier habits to slow weight gain until height catches up, rather than trying to make the child lose weight. An overweight child should never be put on a restrictive diet to lose weight. Restrictive eating can lead to lack of important nutrients that are extremely necessary during the growing years. The wiser choice is to reduce portion sizes, decrease excessive snacks, and build a healthier lifestyle.

Offering children a wide variety of wholesome grain products, fruits and vegetables, low-fat dairy products, lean meats, poultry, fish, eggs, and beans is key. (Refer to the Food Guide Pyramid for specific food choices, recommended daily servings, and portion sizes.) Snacks should be included, too, throughout the day, but they should be selected from nutrient-dense foods rather than empty-calorie choices. And, to balance food intake, physical fitness must be part of daily activity.

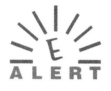

**ALERT**

A child should never be put on a restrictive diet to lose weight. Doing so can result in delayed growth. Instead, healthier habits should be stressed to slow a child's weight gain while waiting for the height to catch up.

## Encouraging Healthier Habits in Children

As a parent, your first course of action should be to support, love, and accept your child for who he or she is. Don't get too caught up on body weight. There are so many other factors in life besides the number found on the bathroom scale. Be as supportive as you can be, and stress the importance of health and healthy eating over being thin and trim. Make note of the ways to do so.

**ESSENTIALS**

All children, regardless of their weight, need love, support, acceptance, and encouragement from their loved ones.

### Keep a Diet Diary for Three to Five Days

Prior to making any dietary changes, keep a log of everything your child eats and drinks for three to five days. This will allow you to estimate and understand where eating problems may be occurring. Also, note physical and sedentary activities and the time your child spends in each. If your child is watching more than an hour and a half of television daily, it may be time to make some changes to his or her activity schedule. Then ask yourself the following questions.

- Is my child eating at least three to five fruits and/or vegetables daily?
- Is my child consuming two servings of milk daily?
- Is my child eating too many desserts or snacks?
- Is my child drinking more than one to two glasses of juice daily?
- How many empty-calorie foods (soft drinks, candies, cookies, pastries) is my child consuming each day?
- Is my child playing video/computer games or watching TV for more than an hour and a half each day?

If you find that your child is not eating recommended servings from each of the food groups and is consuming too many foods with no nutritional value, or that your child is not getting enough activity, it is now time to make some changes. If you find it difficult to manage these concerns yourself, seek professional assistance from a registered dietitian, or ask your doctor for a referral.

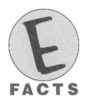

**FACTS**

The number of overweight children in our country has risen by 50 percent in the past decade. One in four children are now classified as overweight or at risk for being overweight.

## Make Better Food Choices

Review the discussion of the Food Guide Pyramid in Chapter 6. Try to incorporate more food choices that fit into the food groups. These choices will help provide a healthier intake of foods without leaving your child feeling deprived. In fact, eating healthier may actually make you and your child feel better overall. Also begin to add more fruit and vegetables, lean meats, low-fat dairy products, whole-grain breads, and complex carbohydrates. Limit high-fat foods, including fried foods, convenience food items, and whole milk products. Reduce empty-calorie snacks and soft drinks, and offer snack options like popcorn, pretzels, dried and fresh fruit, graham crackers, fresh vegetable sticks, and low-fat yogurt.

## Avoid Restriction of Any Particular Food

If your child loves to eat chocolate chip cookies, then allow these in moderation. By restricting any one or two foods, you make that food more desirable. Offer options like small cookies or treats but only once a day, for example. You can also remove unhealthy foods from the house and replace them with better options. If there aren't any potato chips available at night, a piece of fruit will be more appealing as a snack.

## Change Unhealthy Behaviors Associated with Eating

Changing unhealthy behaviors—for example, not allowing food to be eaten in front of the television or away from the kitchen table—can help in improving bad eating behaviors. Changing these habits and food behaviors will help in determining how hungry your child really is. If your child really wants that dish of ice cream, then she must sit down at the table to eat it. If your child doesn't want to give up a favorite TV program, then he really doesn't want that dish of ice cream that badly after all.

## Limit Dining Out

Cutting back on eating out, especially fast-food eating, is key to improving overall healthy food habits. Eating out is a part of the American culture, but too much can wreak havoc on one's daily calorie and fat intake. Large portion sizes, fried foods, and high-fat selections can all contribute to overeating and increase the risk of a child's becoming overweight. You can still eat out, just with healthier options, especially when feeding kids. Try to limit eating out to no more than two to three times each week, and compromise with your children to make good food choices. Here are some ideas on how to do so:

- Choose a plain hamburger kid's meal with low-fat milk.
- Share French fries with someone else.
- Try applesauce as a substitute for French fries, if available.
- Incorporate an occasional salad with low-fat dressing.
- Opt for a stuffed baked potato for a change.

- Order plain cheese thin-crust pizza over stuffed versions.
- Try a sub sandwich, without added mayonnaise or sauce.
- Choose baked chicken sandwiches over fried.

## Keep Active

Parents should encourage activity for all children, regardless of their weight. The benefits associated with active lifestyles are numerous at all stages of life. By enjoying active lifestyles during their early years, children will grow up with an appreciation for healthier lives. Encourage team sports and group programs. Get involved with your child. Do things together. Activities like walking, biking, swimming, skating, sledding, boating, and bowling are just some of the many ways to keep yourself active and have fun as well.

## Stop Feeding Emotions with Food

Many of the reasons that adults eat are associated with boredom, loneliness, and stress. Kids often eat for similar reasons. Don't raise your children to follow this pattern. Have you ever seen a parent hand a child a cookie or lollipop to stop crying or offer ice cream to a child who is bored? All of a sudden the child stops crying or feels fulfilled. Did the food solve the problem associated with the crying or boredom or just temporarily cover it up until the next time? Behaviors such as these often lead to a lifelong habit of feeding emotions with food, a habit that many adults find difficult to break.

## Understand Your Responsibilities as a Parent

Parents are responsible for feeding their children from the early years and teaching them good eating habits. Young children are responsible for eating the foods offered to them. Their parents hope that as the children grow, they will take on additional responsibilities for making good food decisions. Parents need to set the stage by being good role models for their children. When good examples are set regarding foods purchased, foods brought into the house, foods served for dinner, snacking, and so forth, children will learn to follow these behaviors.

**FACTS**

You cannot force your child to eat. He'll eat when he is hungry and stop when he is full. But you can be a good role model and a good teacher.

# Building Positive Body Image in Your Child

In this world of superhunks and flawless supermodels, it is difficult for children to grow up believing that they will not be built this way. When growth patterns do not necessary follow suit during the preteen and teen years, it is hard to understand that these idealistic shapes are the exception rather than the norm. Many people still base their self-worth on their size and shape.

At toddler and preschool ages, many children are built alike, but changes suddenly occur during the elementary and middle-school years. There is no way of telling how and when each child's final growth spurt will take place. Obviously many of the factors relating to a child's growth are genetic. Taller parents usually have children who are taller, and shorter parents usually have shorter children. But genetics are not always to blame. The environment in which one lives can significantly contribute to one's weight. Families who eat and snack frequently raise children who do the same. Active parents usually raise active children. And just as overeating habits can be mimicked, so can dieting habits. Mothers who constantly follow trendy fad diets demonstrate to their children that these are appropriate behaviors for them, too. Parents need to understand how and what they transfer to their children's behaviors.

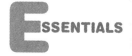

**SSENTIALS**

Raising children to have a positive body image, self-confidence, and self-esteem is just as important in raising healthy children as the foods they choose.

The media also has a great influence on body image. Children as young as eight years of age are now concerned about their weight. The pressure to be "popular" and "fit in" with the "popular crowd" is often centered on how a person looks. But the factor that is often overlooked is how a person feels. A good self-image often projects as self-confidence. It can make a person look better overall and be much more important in the long run than how a person looks on the outside.

## Are You Passing Your Behaviors on to Your Child?

Think about how you feel about your body. Does your body image influence your child's body image as well? Do you feel you have a positive or negative body image? Ask yourself these questions:

- Do I constantly comment about my size and shape?
- Do I often indicate that I am too short, too fat, or not shaped as well as another person?
- Do I judge myself according to my clothes size?

If you responded yes to these questions, you are spending too much time and energy worrying about your size and shape. These behaviors *do* influence your children's attitudes, too. This constant obsession with negative body image has a strong impact on self-esteem. They can impact other areas of life including relationships with others, career, and family life.

## Be Accepting and Nurturing

People need to learn to accept themselves and others for who they are. They should aim to be the best they can be. They need to emphasize positive assets, avoid discrimination against themselves, and set examples for those around them based on who they are rather than how they look. Accepting yourself is the first step toward accepting others. By doing so you will learn to share this behavior with future generations and live a better life overall.

Parents of overweight children need to nurture their children properly. They need to demonstrate their love and support no matter what size or shape their child is. Yes, it is important to aim for healthy food choices and do what you can for overall health, but it's also important to encourage your child to be the best he or she can be. Not everyone can be tall and slim. Feeling loved and being secure is so much more important than just fitting into a smaller size. Demonstrate your positive behaviors to your child, and your child will likely be a better person for it.

# Establishing Good Habits You Can Live With

Set goals for yourself and your family. Sit down if you need to and plan out a course of action. Begin with some rules. Try to turn these into future habits. You'll be surprised how much better you will feel.

## Set Regular Meal and Snack Times

Families who eat regularly tend to eat more healthfully. Planning regular meals helps in selecting a greater variety of foods and serving balanced food choices. It is difficult to get the entire family together for a sit-down meal each night, but planning to do so on several nights a week will encourage family members to plan their schedules accordingly. Make the meal fun, too. Let various members of the family either prepare or plan their favorite meals. It lessens the load of work on any one person and provides a greater chance for families to communicate and enjoy each other's company, too.

## Seek out New Recipes

If you have a recipe file that hasn't been used in years, throw it out and start over. Look for recipes the entire family will enjoy and get the family involved in shopping and preparing them as well. Look in newspapers and magazines and talk to friends about their favorite new recipes. You may find that this will be fun for you as well.

## Keep an Ongoing Shopping List and Shop Weekly

Planning properly, keeping lists of needed foods, and shopping regularly all keep families on track with stocking staples, being able to prepare quick and healthy meals, and avoiding impulse eating. Place a blank pad of paper on the kitchen counter or attach one to the refrigerator with a magnet. Encourage family members to jot down foods and supplies that need to be purchased. If you have the items on hand, preparing meals is so much easier and less stressful in the long run.

## Prepare Extra Foods on the Weekend

Prepare greater amounts of food over the weekend when you have more time and save these for busier nights. Take advantage of extra time to prepare larger quantities of main dishes or special foods, like banana breads or yogurt pies, that can more easily be served during hectic weekdays.

## Pack Snacks to Go

Make up portions of snacks that are easily portable, and be sure to keep them handy. If you find yourself constantly carpooling your child around during the day and hunger pangs strike, keep snacks available in the car, in backpacks, or for after-school activities.

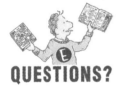

**QUESTIONS?**

**What are some good snacks to pack for eating on the go?**
Dried fruits, trail mixes, nuts, granola bars, cheese sticks, pudding cups, pretzels, and 100 percent juice drinks are good to have on hand. They can easily be taken in the car or packed in a backpack for a quick treat.

## Identify Problem Times of the Day

Identify your child's problem eating times, and try to find alternate activities. If your child (or yourself) is guilty of eating in front of the television at night or snacking inappropriately after school, try to rearrange schedules. Plan activities during those times like sports practices or taking a walk during long television periods, or set out preplanned snack choices after school. Kids who grab snacks after school often choose the first food they see. Placing fresh fruit or a bowl of popcorn on the table will encourage a healthier snack choice than in the contents of the cookie jar.

## Make Time for Activities

Schedule activity time just like you schedule dance class or an appointment. Encouraging a wind-down period, like taking a walk after dinner for fifteen minutes or so, will allow time to relax and open lines of communication with the entire family.

## Be Wise When Eating Out

If possible, monitor your eating out of the house. Try to limit eating away from home to no more than two or three times each week. Eating out can encourage high-fat calorie consumption. Be wise with food selections at restaurants. Avoid fast foods when possible. When you do eat out, choose restaurants that offer a variety of healthier choices.

**E**SSENTIALS

The best approach to handling an overweight child is through a combined long-term approach to weight management and physical activity.

No one chooses to be overweight, particularly a child. As parents, it is up to us to manage any weight-related problem before it becomes uncontrollable. By setting a good example ourselves, we can take the first step in nurturing and nourishing our future generations. Being supportive, loving, and caring is as important as feeding our children a healthy variety of foods. In doing so, we can set the stage for raising healthier children. Doesn't this make good sense?

## CHAPTER 14
# *Fitting In Fitness*

Did you know that a regular exercise program is the most effective way to lose and maintain weight? The benefits don't just come from programs and equipment found in health clubs and from using expensive machines. Exercise is achieved from any activity that gets you moving, whether it is walking the dog, gardening, cleaning house, or playing with your kids.

# The Truth about Exercise

What do you know about exercise and physical fitness? Let's test you. Answer the following true-or-false questions:

1. In order to reap the benefits of exercise you need to push yourself to your limits.
2. If you sweat more, you lose more weight.
3. Exercising will make you eat more overall.
4. The best option for losing weight would include a combination of aerobic conditioning and strength training.
5. It doesn't pay to begin an exercise program as a senior citizen if you have never exercised before in your life.
6. Spot reducing is the best way to tackle a problem with fat on a particular part of the body.
7. Cellulite is more difficult to lose than body fat.

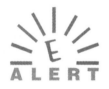

**ALERT**

People of all sizes, shapes, and of all ages can reap the benefits of physical activity.

Here are the answers:

1. **False.** You will be relieved to know that excessive exercise can actually do more harm than good. Pushing yourself too hard increases risk of injuries to the bones, joints, and muscles and can also make you dislike exercising altogether. You would benefit more from slowing it down, enjoying what you are doing, and making exercise a part of your everyday routine.
2. **False.** Water weight can be lost through excess perspiration and can reduce the number on the scale, but this is only temporary. Once fluids are reintroduced to the body, this water weight will return. Any person who is exercising should replace fluids on a regular basis.
3. **False.** It is true that some people do experience variations in their appetite, but on the whole regular exercise should not increase appetite, nor should it decrease it.

4. **True.** People tend to lose weight more quickly and effectively when incorporating both aerobics and strength training into their regular exercise routine. Aerobic activities do burn more calories overall, but strength training builds more muscle, which burns more calories than body fat.

5. **False.** Evidence has shown that people of all ages can benefit from an exercise program. Even something as simple as a regular walking program can be of great benefit. By getting involved in a regular fitness routine, individuals can gain muscle mass and improve strength, flexibility, and endurance. Individuals with elevated blood pressures and who suffer from elevated blood sugar levels as a result of noninsulin-dependent diabetes can even reduce their levels by incorporating an exercise routine and losing several pounds.

6. **False.** Doing just sit-ups to trim a flabby stomach or leg presses to slim the thighs is not the best course of action. Spot-reducing attempts just don't work overall. The best way to lose that flabby stomach or trim those thighs is to build muscles throughout the entire body with a regular fitness program while cutting excess fat and calories at the same time. Burning off those extra calories will help reduce the spots along with other troublesome parts of the body too.

7. **False.** Cellulite and body fat are one and the same. Cellulite is just fat with that awful dimply appearance, which comes from the way it is deposited in the body. Again, weight loss through a plan of reduced calories and fat and an increase in exercise will help combat that extra cellulite and fat.

# The Benefits of Physical Activity

Exercise and a planned physical fitness program are important. Exercise or physical fitness and activities of all types contribute to an active lifestyle. The more you move, the healthier you are.

In other words, a person with high blood pressure can lower his blood pressure, and an overweight person can lose weight. A depressed person can even begin to feel better. Isn't it worth the effort?

It doesn't matter where or how you begin. There are many types of activities you can do to help you change your sedentary lifestyle into a more active one. You can join an aerobics or step class; go biking, swimming, jogging, skiing, skating, or even dancing; or learn a team sport like tennis, softball, football, or basketball. If you like, you can just walk your dog around the block. Any and all activities add up. Determine what you like to do and build a daily program from that.

## Weight Loss and Maintenance

Physical activity helps a person lose weight by burning additional calories that otherwise could be stored as fat in the body. A person's body weight is regulated by the number of calories consumed. When more calories are consumed than are used for energy, weight gain occurs. When more calories are burned for energy than are consumed, weight loss occurs. Balancing calories that are consumed with calories that are burned results in weight maintenance.

Any type of activity you choose will help in burning up extra calories. Some may be more effective in weight loss than others. Strenuous activities like running, dancing, and biking help burn more calories than more moderate activities like walking and gardening. But it all adds up. See how your favorite activity ranks in the chart below. To calculate the approximate number of calories burned from each activity, multiply the number listed by your weight and then by the number of minutes spent doing each activity.

| ACTIVITY | APPROXIMATE CALORIES/MINUTE |
| --- | --- |
| Dancing, aerobic | 0.077 |
| Dancing, ballroom | 0.023 |
| Fishing | 0.029 |
| Gardening | 0.036 |
| Lawn croquet | 0.026 |
| Mopping floors | 0.028 |
| Mowing grass | 0.051 |

| ACTIVITY | APPROXIMATE CALORIES/MINUTE |
|---|---|
| Playing piano | 0.018 |
| Playing drums | 0.035 |
| Raking leaves | 0.025 |
| Running, 8 minute/mile | 0.100 |
| Running, 6 minute/mile | 0.127 |
| Scrubbing floors | 0.049 |
| Shoveling snow | 0.060 |
| Sitting/reading | 0.010 |
| Swimming, fast | 0.073 |
| Swimming, slow | 0.059 |
| Yard volleyball | 0.044 |
| Walking leisurely | 0.036 |
| Walking up hills | 0.055 |
| Washing car | 0.026 |

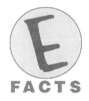

**FACTS**

Over 90 percent of successful dieters incorporate regular exercise into their lifestyle.

Let's say a 150-pound person wants to know how many calories were burned in a sixty-minute walk. Multiply 150 (for weight) times .036 (for activity) times 60 (for minutes spent exercising). The result tells us that 324 calories were burned.

## Heart Health

Routine physical activity helps in reducing risks associated with heart disease and stroke by strengthening the heart muscles, improving blood flow and circulation, increasing high-density lipoprotein levels (HDL—the good cholesterol), and decreasing low-density lipoprotein levels (LDL—the bad cholesterol).

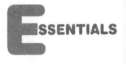 Several ounces of cool water should be consumed every twenty minutes during exercise. If the weather conditions are warm, water should be consumed every ten to fifteen minutes.

## Blood Pressure and Diabetes Control

Incorporating exercise in daily living is effective in controlling blood pressure and noninsulin-dependent diabetes. Even the loss of a few pounds can benefit and reduce one's blood pressure and prevent or control diabetes.

## Builds Stronger Bones and Muscles

Regular physical fitness programs that include weight-bearing activities help build stronger bones and muscles. Continuation of these activities through the years helps maintain bone strength and reduce incidence of bone injuries and fractures.

**E**SSENTIALS Regular exercise is also effective in preventing bone loss that can contribute to osteoporosis in later life.

## Reduction of Bone, Joint, and Back Pain

People with problems relating to bone, joint, and back pain can also benefit from a regular exercise program. Strengthening of muscles, building endurance, and increasing flexibility all assist in improving conditions relating to the bones, joints, and back.

## Better Sleep

Regular exercise allows people to relax more easily and sleep better at night. People who exercise on a regular basis usually have less difficulty falling asleep at night, and once they do so enjoy a more restful and peaceful sleep.

### Increase in Energy Levels

Although some people may believe incorporating exercise in daily activities can be tiresome, it results in just the opposite effect. People who do exercise regularly indicate that they have improved daily energy sources that help them feel better.

### Psychological Improvements

It is a fact that regular exercisers are also ones who feel better about themselves, have greater self-confidence, and are less likely to be depressed. These individuals are also better able to handle stress in their daily lives.

### Increased Social Opportunities

Joining an exercise class, fitness club, golf foursome, tennis league, or sports team offers many opportunities to meet people, enjoy the company of others, and keep active. Be a team player and see how much you can gain.

**E**SSENTIALS  Regular exercise keeps energy levels up, reduces overall stress, and adds to a general feeling of physical and emotional well-being.

## What Kind of Exercise Should I Do?

There are many types of activities available to you. Obviously whatever you choose, you should enjoy. But some exercises offer greater benefits than others do.

### Aerobic Conditioning

Aerobic activity is one type of activity that helps your heart work harder and become more efficient over the long run. The primary goal of an aerobic activity is to increase the heart and breathing rates (still to safe levels) for an extended period of time. To gain the maximum benefits from an aerobic activity, these activities should be completed a minimum of three times per week. They should be repeated for a length of time of approximately twenty to thirty minutes, where large muscle groups are moving at an even pace. Examples of aerobic activities include jogging, fast walking, biking, dancing, skating, and skiing. While performing an aerobic activity, you will breathe harder during the time your heart is working harder. It is important to monitor your heart rate to determine how effective your workout really is. Later in the chapter you will learn how to determine your target heart rate and evaluate yourself.

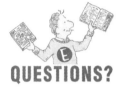

**QUESTIONS?**

**What is the difference between aerobic and anaerobic activity?**
Aerobic means "with oxygen" and denotes activities where oxygen demand can be met continuously during performance, such as walking or jogging. Anaerobic means "without oxygen" and denotes activities where the muscles are using oxygen faster than the heart and lungs can deliver it. These activities include quick stop-and-go movements, like in football, baseball, and tennis.

## Everyday Moderate Activities

Other activities that are not necessarily considered aerobic are those that are more moderate in intensity. These include activities such as gardening, cleaning house, raking leaves, mowing the grass, playing with children, and leisure walking. Although these activities may not assist in initially losing weight, they are just as important as aerobic activities for overall health and weight maintenance. Accumulation of several of these types of activities adds up to more calories burned overall. Incorporating more of these types of activities on a daily basis can lead to a more active lifestyle, keep boredom at bay, and help eliminate excess consumption of foods, too. Additional fitness benefits are gained for individuals who accumulate at least thirty minutes of moderate activities each day.

## Strengthening Exercises

Exercises that include weight bearing and weight training should be as much of a part of your exercise routine as aerobic conditioning. These types of activities help strengthen muscles and bones; improve overall conditioning, endurance and overall balance; and assist in preventing injuries. Strength-training exercises should be incorporated into regular exercise programs at least twice per week.

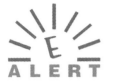

Muscle weighs more than fat, so building up muscle can initially add several pounds rather than taking them off, but in time this will reverse.

## Flexibility Exercises

Exercises that improve flexibility are those that help to move your joints in all areas of motion, like stretching exercises. Improved flexibility allows individuals to move their bodies more freely and prevent injuries to the muscles that control movement of the joints of the shoulders, knees, elbows, hips, and ankles. Stretching exercises should be incorporated into your regular fitness routine. Stretching helps elongate the muscles and connective tissues that prevent stiffness in the body. When you stretch, hold these stretches for twenty to thirty seconds or as long as you can. Try stretching whenever you can—in front of the television, in your car, during a coffee break, or at the gym. You should also stretch after strength-training exercises for maximum benefits.

## How Much Should I Exercise?

Most experts agree that every person should incorporate twenty to thirty minutes of aerobic activity into their daily lives, three or more times each week, along with a program of muscle conditioning and strengthening at least two times each week.

Are you meeting recommended daily requirements? Or do you consider yourself more of a computer-couch potato? We are all guilty of it at times, and there's nothing wrong with occasional inactivity. Sitting on the couch or in front of the computer keeps your body sedentary and at a low activity level. It might do your mind some good, but it doesn't do much for your body. Try these tips for adding more movement into your otherwise lazy body.

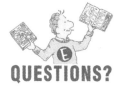

**What time of the day is best to exercise?**
There is no specific time of day that is more beneficial than another—whatever works best for your schedule is best for you. Most people do prefer to exercise first thing in the morning, as this allows them to "get it over with" in case other duties or tiredness sets in later in the day or evening.

While watching TV, do the following stretches and/or exercises:

- Sit on the floor and stretch your legs and arms (without bouncing).
- Ride a stationary bike, walk on a treadmill, step up and down, or just walk in place.
- Jump rope or run in place during commercials.

While working on the computer:

- Stretch, flex, and point your legs, feet, and toes.
- Reach your arms as high as you can every fifteen minutes or after each typed page.
- Roll your shoulders, turning your head from side to side.
- Stretch and massage your fingers and palms every thirty minutes or so.

These activities don't take the place of an active lifestyle, but they surely can help.

## Getting Started on Your Exercise Program

Every exercise program should begin with a plan. Whether you decide to work out in a gym or start a walking program, the best success lies with a program that is incorporated into daily schedules. You need to be committed, motivated, and also enjoy what you are doing in order to gain benefits over the long haul.

## Evaluate Your Health

If you have not had a recent physical examination or are over the age of sixty, you should see your doctor before you begin a regular fitness program. It is always a wise idea. Your doctor can determine if you have any health-related problems that need to be observed, such as heart problems, chest pains, high blood pressure, diabetes, or arthritis.

## Begin Slowly

Don't be in such a rush. Don't try too much too soon. Start gradually and work your way up, especially if you have not been exercising previously. This will allow your body to adjust to the changes that hopefully will be continued for a long time to come.

## Get Your Gear

Select shoes that are appropriate for the activity you choose, and make sure they fit. There are no longer just sneakers to buy. Seek out the right type for your activity and your feet. Find clothes that work, too. If you are walking or jogging outdoors, buy layers that can be added with weather changes. If you choose indoor activities, buy loose, comfortable styles.

When you're buying sneakers, keep in mind the following suggestions:

- Try on several different brands and sizes before making a selection.
- Shop later in the day, after a workout, when swelling will make your feet slightly larger.
- Try shoes on with appropriate athletic socks. Tie them snugly, too.
- Make sure both shoes fit. Sometimes one foot may be slightly larger than the other.
- Walk around in the store before you buy. Don't make a rash decision that you may regret later.

## Choose Activities You Enjoy

An exercise routine is good only if it's followed regularly. You should enjoy what you do. Try a dance class or join a walking group. Choose whatever you like, whatever keeps you going. Try watching television while walking on a treadmill or while pedaling on a stationary bike. Or read a juicy novel.

**E**SSENTIALS

Boredom is the number one reason many people stop exercising. If your exercise routine is too boring, find something else.

## Make a Schedule

Just as you should plan your meals and snacks, it is important to plan your activities. Put fitness dates on the calendar just like you would do for a meeting or appointment. Set up times for tennis, biking, walking, or just working around the house. This helps keep you on track from day to day.

## Alternate Your Routine

Select from a variety of activities you enjoy to avoid boredom over the long run. If you walk or bike regularly, choose different routes for a change. If you go to a fitness club, try different group classes or equipment on different days of the week.

## Find a Friend

People who exercise with others find their workouts more exciting and fun. Friends (and family members) who join efforts offer encouragement to keep you motivated. And what a great way to visit with others!

## Challenge Yourself

It's essential to set goals, both short- and long-term goals, just like you do with eating behaviors. These goals will offer you the challenge and inspiration you need to keep going. And they can be fun to accomplish, too.

# Starting a Walking Program

Many people find walking the most suitable form of exercise. It does not require any special equipment, does not cost anything, and can be enjoyed any time of year both indoors and outdoors. Walking has been shown to be the most popular form of exercise, too—it makes people feel more energized, improves heart rates, and helps reduce body fat. It is also highly enjoyed when accompanied by family members, friends, or even with the family dog.

Walking at a steady but moderate pace is suggested for achieving the greatest benefits. Walking too slow does not raise one's heart rate as effectively as walking at a brisker level, but it still offers improved fitness levels, particularly for people who are just beginning an exercise routine.

Proper walking form includes the following elements:

- Keeping your back straight and head erect.
- Keeping your toes pointed straight ahead.
- Letting your arms swing loosely at your sides, with elbows bent at about 90 degree angles.
- Landing on your heels first, then rolling foot forward to move off of the balls of your feet.

People who may be enthusiastic about their walking program may wish to monitor their mileage and increase it over time. Attaching a pedometer to your waistband may be one helpful motivator. This small tool offers information regarding miles and number of steps walked. Some even calculate calories burned as well. You can also plan your walking routes and use the odometer on your car to determine the distance you have covered. In any case, a walking program should be one that is started slowly and increased over time for maximum benefits. Here is a sample program that may work for you.

| WEEK | WARM-UP | BRISK WALKING | COOL DOWN |
|------|---------|---------------|-----------|
| 1 | 5 minutes | 5 minutes | 5 minutes |
| 2 | 5 minutes | 7 minutes | 5 minutes |
| 3 | 5 minutes | 9 minutes | 5 minutes |
| 4 | 5 minutes | 11 minutes | 5 minutes |
| 5 | 5 minutes | 13 minutes | 5 minutes |
| 6 | 5 minutes | 15 minutes | 5 minutes |
| 7 | 5 minutes | 18 minutes | 5 minutes |
| 8 | 5 minutes | 20 minutes | 5 minutes |
| 9 | 5 minutes | 23 minutes | 5 minutes |
| 10 | 5 minutes | 25 minutes | 5 minutes |
| 11 | 5 minutes | 28 minutes | 5 minutes |
| 12 | 5 minutes | 30 minutes | 5 minutes |

Warming up before beginning any exercise prepares your heart and other muscles for the work that will be required from them. This warm-up should last for about five minutes at a slow pace. A gradual increase can then follow.

The cool-down period should last for about five minutes. This will allow the heart rate to decline at an appropriate rate. Walking at a slow pace is appropriate as a cool-down, similar to the warm-up.

## What about Fluids?

Exercise of any type and in all weather conditions causes fluid loss through perspiration. Athletes of all abilities should compensate for this loss by consuming plenty of fluids before and during their workouts.

Many athletes opt for sports drinks to replace their fluids. Sport drinks really offer little benefit for the average to moderate athlete who is exercising for an hour and a half or less at a time, but they can be beneficial to more competitive athletes. Sports drinks include additional carbohydrates, primarily as sugar, and calories, which the average athlete does not necessarily need.

# Measuring Your Heart Rate

Checking your heart rate or counting your pulse rate during activity periods allows you to monitor the effect that the activity is having on your heart. You can do this in several ways. Taking your pulse allows you to count the number of times your heart beats. Try doing this by gently placing your index and middle fingers—don't use your thumb, as it has its own pulse— either on your wrist or neck. While watching the second hand on a clock, count the number of beats for fifteen seconds. Multiply this number by four to determine the number of beats per minute. Use the chart in **FIGURE 14-2** to determine how you rate.

**FIGURE 14-2:** Target heart rate chart

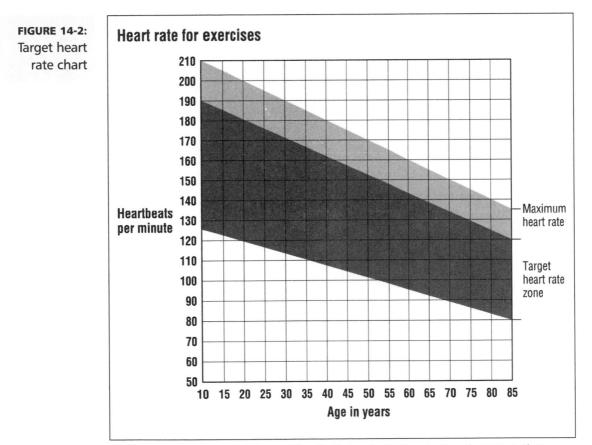

Adapted from *Nutrition and Fitness: Lifestyle Choices for Wellness* by Dorothy F. West, Ph.D. Tinley Park, IL: Goodheart-Willcox, 2000.

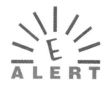

A general rule for replenishing thirst after a workout is to drink enough to satisfy thirst, then drink some more. A person's thirst mechanism is not a good indication of their body's need for fluids, and drinking the extra fluid allows for sufficient intake.

You can also manually calculate your target heart rate zone. To do so, you must first determine your maximum heart rate by subtracting your age from 220. For example, if you are forty years old, your maximum heart rate would be 180 (220 minus 40). Then calculate your target heart rate zone. This is usually 60 to 75 percent of the maximum heart rate for most people, especially those who have not regularly been exercising over the last six months to a year. If you are just beginning to exercise on a regular basis, start with 50 to 60 percent and then work your way up. If this is the case, you should aim for a target heart rate of between 108 to 135 beats per minute. Working within this range will allow most people to improve their overall health and cardiovascular fitness while helping them lose and maintain body weight. Moving beyond this target rate is recommended only for very fit and very active individuals.

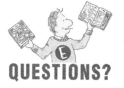

**How much fluid should I drink while exercising?**
Recommendations regarding fluid replacements for exercises that last sixty minutes or less are to drink a minimum of two cups of cool water about two hours prior to exercise and to drink several ounces every ten to twenty minutes during exercise to replace fluids lost through perspiration.

With any aerobic activity, you should aim to exercise within a safe target heart rate zone. This zone is the range in which your heart is obtaining an effective workout. Varying with ages and fitness abilities, this zone is a range between a person's resting heart rate and their maximum heart rate. When you first begin a fitness program, aim for the lower end of your zone, then seek to increase it as your ability increases.

# Exercise Motivators

We all find excuses to avoid exercise. We're either too tired, too busy, or we just don't feel like getting sweaty. Whatever the case may be, exercise should take priority in your life. It shouldn't be considered an optional activity but a necessary one. Find what motivators work for you. If you find that early morning times work better because you're too tired at night, then aim for an activity in the morning. Or if weekends offer better opportunities for a tennis game, then plan for one then.

Here are several helpful motivators that may also work for you:

- Exercise with a friend. Set similar goals and work together to accomplish them.
- Set goals. Make short-term and long-term goals and challenge yourself. Focus on certain goals for each and every day.
- Gain the support of your family and friends. Their encouragement will help you succeed.
- Join a class. Signing up for a class keeps you interested and motivated, and others become dependent on your attendance.
- Log your success. Keep a chart of your plans and successes. It helps keep you challenged.
- Listen to music or a favorite radio talk show. Keeping your mind off of the exercise routine makes the time go by faster.
- Find a group sport. Try something new or something you enjoyed in the past. How about joining a volleyball team, tennis or racquetball match, or even swim aerobics.

Exercise of all types should be part of your everyday lifestyle, just like getting dressed, taking a shower, or eating breakfast. The benefits of a regular program far outweigh the problems associated with lack of physical activity. Each and every activity adds up to your benefit. Now that you understand why you need to incorporate a program into your daily routine, there's no reason to put it off any longer. Start now and make your life and your future better in every way.

## CHAPTER 15
# *Eating Out*

How many times have you tried to dine at your favorite restaurant only to find out that the wait is more than an hour? Or decided to grab your children a quick, fast-food meal and had to wait behind numerous cars at the drive-through window? Have you ever asked yourself if people really eat at home anymore?

## Why We Eat Away from Home

Changes in the American lifestyle over the past few decades have also impacted the trends toward eating out. People are busier than ever before. Schedules are crazier than ever before. And people are making more money than ever before. Family meals are no longer what they used to be. No longer do dads come home by 6:00 p.m. to their family and a hot meal waiting at the table. No longer do moms stay home planning and preparing their evening meals. And no longer do children have open schedules during the dinnertime hour.

Trends today demonstrate that breakfast and lunches are rarely eaten at home, and if they are, they are rarely eaten together as a family. Breakfast meals are traditionally quick and easy and grabbed on the way out the door. Lunches are typically packed or picked up at work, school, or at the corner diner. And dinner? Well, that's up for grabs in most families, depending on the day of the week. Weekends do offer a little extra time, and many families do find some time together at mealtime.

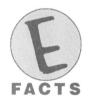

**FACTS**

The frequency of eating out has risen by more than 66 percent in the last two decades. Current estimates are than Americans eat more than a quarter of total meals out of the house.

Eating out serves as a solution to busy households. It may be convenient and fast, but what is it doing to our eating habits? What are restaurant foods doing to our efforts to lose and manage our weight? Does anybody even cook anymore?

## Weight Control and Maintenance Challenges

Eating out can be challenging both for the individual who wants to obtain a nutritional meal and for the person who is trying to lose and maintain weight. Restaurant choices are abundant. And portion sizes, fat, and calories are abundant as well. Serving sizes most commonly found in restaurants truly exceed those standard serving sizes recommended for most foods. It is not uncommon to see a serving for one meal measure at four times that recommended in the Food Guide Pyramid. A typical 3-ounce hamburger patty, ½ cup pasta, or 1 tablespoon of salad dressing (recommended serving sizes) are not considered appropriate serving sizes in most restaurants. In fact, most people would be upset to receive portions of these sizes as they often feel they are not getting what they paid for.

| INSTEAD OF THIS . . . | CHOOSE THIS . . . | SAVE . . . (APPROXIMATE CALORIES) | SAVE . . . (APPROXIMATE GRAMS OF FAT) |
|---|---|---|---|
| Double cheeseburger | plain hamburger | 270 | 10 |
| Supersize french fries | small french fries | 330 | 16 |
| 32-oz. regular soft drink | 12-oz. diet soft drink | 310 | 0 |
| Fried chicken patty sandwich | broiled/grilled chicken fillet sandwich | 160 | 14 |
| 1 slice thick-crust pepperoni pizza | 1 slice thin-crust cheese pizza | 101 | 9 |
| Tuna salad sub sandwich (6-inch) | turkey sub sandwich (6-inch) | 253 | 28 |
| Taco salad with shell | taco salad, no shell | 420 | 31 |

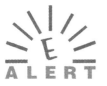

Americans spend more money combined on fast foods alone than they do on higher education, personal computers, or new cars—more than $110 billion a year.

# Healthy Choices in and Around Town

Trends toward eating out are not going to stop. Restaurants, whether they are American, Mexican, Chinese, Italian, Thai, Japanese, pizza, or even fast food can be found anywhere and everywhere you go. Popular chain restaurants help you make familiar selections when you travel, and busy lifestyles are going to continue to keep us grabbing foods on the run. So in order to do your best with the options you have, I will offer you some suggestions on managing your food intake while eating in and around town.

## Monitor the Times You Eat Out

Eating out should be a treat not a regular occurrence, especially for those watching their food intake. You have less control over what goes into your foods, and it's difficult to keep track of those extra calories and larger portions. Plan for those times each week when you want to eat out.

During the week, plan to pack yourself one or two breakfasts or lunches instead of eating out every day. This can help you control your intake at least for those days. Also plan for your adventures out, just like you plan other activities. This will make eating out more fun and keep it from being just another habit.

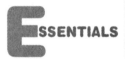

For most people, eating out occasionally will not cause a problem with a healthy lifestyle. It all depends on what is ordered and what is eaten.

## Select Restaurants That Offer Choices

There are so many restaurants available to you. If you can make the choice, do so with care. If there are occasions when someone else makes the choice, be careful in your ordering. In any case, choose restaurants that offer a wide variety of foods and preparation methods. Ask servers about how the food is cooked. If it is not to your liking, speak to the chef about making a special request. Remember, you are a paying customer. You should get what you ask for and pay for.

## Make Healthy Menu Selections

Look for menu items that are lower in fat. Stay away from fried, batter-dipped, and creamy foods. Ask for substitutions for french fries, hash browns, or potato chips. Restaurants are very willing to provide fresh fruit and vegetable replacements. Order salad with the dressing on the side. Order turkey or roast beef with the gravy on the side. This way you can control how much is poured on top. Baked potatoes should be ordered plain instead of stuffed with butter and sour cream. Watch the bread basket, too. Eating a breadstick or a roll before a sandwich can double or triple the amount of bread you may want to consume at one meal. Also, keep away from that extra butter or margarine. It adds up quickly.

## Watch Your Portions

Many people like to be served big portions in restaurants because they feel they get what they pay for. But is more really better? Just because that fish or chicken dish is delicious doesn't mean you need to finish it off all at once. Take some home for another meal. How about removing half before you even start eating?

If you put half away in a doggie bag before you start to eat, it is unlikely that you will open the bag again while you're still at the table. Out of sight, out of mind. But if you keep picking at the meal, it is likely that you will consume it all in one sitting. Is this really good for you?

**ALERT**

You don't need to belong to the "clean your plate club'" when eating out. No one expects you to finish every bite on your plate.

Some meals are actually up to four to six times the recommended serving size. Is this what you want to eat? Understanding and practicing portion control is difficult, but it gets easier as time goes on. If you like, you can even share your meal with someone else. Many restaurants even encourage sharing.

## Try Desserts Occasionally

And, oh yes, desserts are tempting. Many people love to finish off their meals with a tasty, sweet dessert. If you feel pressured into dessert, seek healthier choices. How about fresh fruit or a fruit sorbet? Or angel food cake topped with fresh strawberries?

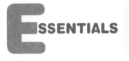

**E**SSENTIALS Most fine restaurants now offer healthy dessert options for their patrons. Just ask!

## The Fast-Food Dilemma

Fast-food dining has become an American pastime, particularly for families with young children. Fast foods are also a solution for a quick meal. Fast-food restaurants are found on practically every corner on every main street in town. Choices are plentiful, served quick, and inexpensive—just what many people want.

Eating at fast-food restaurants is within the realm of possibility. You don't have to avoid them altogether. Just limit the number of times you eat at them, and be sure to balance fast-food meals with other foods lower in fat and calories throughout the day.

In order to keep your diet in line, stay away from double burgers, double cheese, bacon, large fries, and supersized beverages. They can offer large-sized problems. Stick with regular or even child-sized portions.

Look for baked or broiled chicken sandwiches, even vegetarian burgers. These have been creeping up on menus everywhere. Add lettuce, tomatoes, and pickles on a whole-grain bun, without the extra mayonnaise, of course, and you can have a healthy sandwich.

Try a sub sandwich once in a while. Sliced turkey or roast beef with shredded lettuce and tomatoes are a good choice.

Limit any food that may be oily, creamy, or full of mayonnaise, like chicken salads, egg salads, tuna salads, and potato salads. These may sound healthy, but the extra oil and mayonnaise added to them makes them very high in fat.

Keep baked potatoes plain. When you add toppings, your potato can become laden with a lot of extra fat and calories. Top with fresh vegetables and maybe some lower-fat cheese.

Salads can be a good choice but also a not-so-good one. Stay away from higher-fat selections like cheese, croutons, sunflower seeds, and higher-fat dressings. Opt for many vegetables and top with a lower-fat dressing. Also beware of taco salads. These can be full of fat and calories. Fried taco shells, guacamole, sour cream, and refried beans can do wonders to adding up unnecessary calories and fat.

Always order sauces on the side. Whether it be the salad dressing or gravy, the barbecue sauce or honey, it's best to add it yourself.

Try lower-fat condiments. Lemon juice, lower-fat salad dressings and mustard offer better choices than higher-fat sauces and dressings.

If you are going out for pizza, opt for the thin crust with vegetables, and if you're daring, ask for lower-fat cheese. Pizza can be loaded with fat if it has stuffed crust, double cheese, sausage, pepperoni, or other high-fat meats.

Choose water, 100 percent fruit juice, or diet soft drinks over regular soft drinks, especially large-sized ones. Twelve ounces of a regular soft drink alone contains 10 teaspoons of sugar. Can you image drinking a 30-ounce beverage, filled with 25 teaspoons of sugar? WOW!

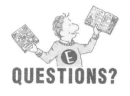

**QUESTIONS?**

**Why is fast food labeled as being so bad?**
Fast food is traditionally labeled as a "not-so-good" choice because many of the foods offered are higher in fat, calories, and sodium. Meals are also notorious for being lower in fiber and vitamins A and C. But fast foods can also be healthy foods. It is possible to make better choices with fast foods. Just be smart with your selections.

Be careful with desserts, especially pies, cookies, and brownies. Choose an occasional small low-fat frozen yogurt cone. These are tasty and not too fattening either.

## Restaurant Choices: Good and Bad

Americans are known for their diverse selection of foods. The interest in ethnic restaurants has grown tremendously over the last decade. People everywhere are continually seeking out the newest and hottest food trends. It's good to know, though, what's good and not-so-good about some of these meal selections. Here is a rundown for you.

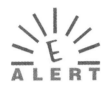

Be careful when adding butter, margarine, sour cream, creamed spinach, and extra cheese to baked potatoes. They can increase calories by as much as 200 to 500 calories per serving.

## American

American grills and family-style restaurants are available to consumers in many different price ranges. These restaurants typically cater to families who opt for a variety of food choices and selections. The large variety of foods found here makes it possible to satisfy everyone's appetite and preferences, too.

Healthier options include the following:

✔ Baked, grilled entrées
✔ Green salads
✔ Broth-based soups
✔ Fruit platters
✔ Vegetarian dishes

Be cautious of these things:

✘ Excess cheese
✘ Fried foods
✘ Batter-dipped fish, chicken, or potatoes
✘ Creamy soups
✘ Toppings on salads, baked potatoes
✘ Extra oil in stir-fries and pastas

Ask the server to do this:

▶ Put salad dressing or gravy on the side
▶ Substitute fruit for potatoes
▶ Provide whole-grain bread over croissants

**E**SSENTIALS   Ask yourself this question, "Would I rather my leftovers go to waste or to my waist?" You decide what's best for them.

## Italian

Italian meals can range from inexpensive to costly, from healthy choices to heavy, high-fat meals. Words like parmigiana, lasagna, alfredo, calamari, white clam sauce, and cannoli often come to mind here. Also beware of extra oil and fat used on appetizers and on pasta dishes. Many Italian restaurants now even serve oil to pour on fresh bread.

For best recommendations here, try sharing menu selections or seek out our healthier options.

Healthier options include the following:

✔ Artichoke hearts
✔ Sun-dried tomatoes
✔ Marinara sauce or tomato-based sauce
✔ Light red sauce
✔ Red or white wine sauce
✔ Light mushroom sauce
✔ Capers, herbs, spices
✔ Garlic and oregano
✔ Florentine
✔ Grilled
✔ Primavera (not cream sauce)
✔ Lemon juice or lemon sauce
✔ Piccata (lemon-wine sauce)
✔ Italian ice

Be cautious of these things:

✗ Alfredo
✗ Butter sauce
✗ Carbonara (butter, eggs, bacon) and creamy sauce
✗ Fried foods

✘ Parmigiana (baked with cheese)
✘ Meats like pancetta, prosciutto, sausage
✘ Oil
✘ Stuffed with cheese
✘ Manicotti, cannelloni, lasagna, ravioli
✘ Creamy desserts, like cannoli

Ask the server to do this:

▶ Hold the bread basket
▶ Put sauce on the side
▶ Use light cheese
▶ Put half in a doggie bag

## Asian

Whether it's Chinese, Japanese, or Thai, Asian restaurants are very popular among Americans today. These foods are often considered healthier choices because of the many fresh vegetables used in cooking. But foods can be low in fat or high in fat, depending on menu selections. Sweet-and-sour foods, tempuras, and fried entrées can be found on many menus. But here again, sharing dishes is an option many people enjoy.

Healthier options include the following:

✔ Steamed chicken, fish, shrimp, seafood, and vegetables
✔ Other steamed, braised, simmered, boiled, broiled dishes
✔ Tofu (bean curd)

Be cautious of these things:

✘ Deep-fried, pan-fried, batter-fried, batter-dipped, or breaded foods
✘ Nuts, like cashews, peanuts
✘ Duck
✘ Crispy noodles
✘ Menu preparations called "golden brown"

✗ Dishes made with coconut milk
✗ Sweet-and-sour dishes
✗ Dishes served in a "bird's nest"
✗ Tempura preparation

Ask the server to do this:

▶ Hold the peanuts, cashews, or crispy noodles
▶ Prepare without MSG
▶ Reduce the oil
▶ Put the dressing or sauce on the side
▶ Substitute chicken for duck

## Deli-Type and Sandwich Shops

Gaining in popularity, delis and sub sandwich shops are being advertised as healthier options to fast-food restaurants. Some foods here can fit that bill, but others do not. Portion sizes are often large, both in the size of the bun and the amount of meat piled on top. Because many sandwiches can be made to order, you have the benefit of making special requests that can help you.

Healthier options include the following:

✔ Whole-grain breads, rolls
✔ Lettuce, tomatoes, pickles
✔ Mustard
✔ Sliced turkey, chicken, ham
✔ Plain tuna, without added mayonnaise
✔ Broth-based soups

Be cautious of these things:

✗ Luncheon meats, like bologna, salami, corned beef, or pastrami
✗ Meatball sandwiches
✗ Sausage and pepperoni
✗ Club sandwiches

✘ Tuna melts
✘ Mayonnaise
✘ Reuben sandwiches
✘ Large portions
✘ Cream-based soups
✘ Potato chips

Ask the server to do this:

▶ Top with lots of fresh vegetables
▶ Serve mayonnaise on the side
▶ Cut sandwich in half to share
▶ Remove chips

## Fast Food

Fast food is found everywhere. Every corner and shopping mall seems to have one type of fast-food restaurant or another. They are even popping up in airports, hospitals, and in local high schools. How can we best eat at them?

Healthier choices include the following:

✔ Grilled chicken sandwiches
✔ Baked potatoes (plain)
✔ Salads (with low-fat dressing)
✔ Single hamburger or kid-sized sandwich
✔ Small fries
✔ Low-fat milk
✔ Low-fat frozen yogurt

Be cautious of these things:

✘ Double burgers, bacon, and extra cheese
✘ Fried chicken and fish sandwiches
✘ Cheese sauce
✘ Croissants

✘ Fried chicken nuggets
✘ Large portions of french fries
✘ Onion rings
✘ Sauces
✘ Extra-large beverages

Ask the server to do this:

▶ Make a plain hamburger
▶ Give you a kid's meal portion
▶ Put no mayonnaise or special sauce on the sandwich

**E**SSENTIALS

High amounts of fast foods in the diet can contribute to obesity. These foods can also put people at risk for coronary heart disease and various types of cancer.

Compare these two fast meals. The first person has a large cheeseburger, a supersize French fries, and a 32-ounce soft drink. The second person has a plain hamburger, small French fries, a side salad with low-fat dressing, and a 12-ounce diet soda. The first person ingests approximately 1,380 calories and 56 grams of fat. The second gets about 555 calories and 19 grams of fat. Quite a difference.

## Mexican

Mexican foods have often been given a bad rap because of the high amount of calories and fat found within them. But there are some good choices for you to make. You just have to be careful with your selections, particularly in fast-food Mexican-style restaurants.

Healthier options include the following:

✔ Salsa
✔ Chili
✔ Enchiladas
✔ Burritos

✔ Fajitas
✔ Gazpacho
✔ Soft tacos, corn or flour tortilla
✔ Lettuce, tomato, onions
✔ Chicken
✔ Spicy beef
✔ Grilled, simmered foods
✔ Lower-fat cheese

Be cautious of these things:

✘ Taco chips, tortilla shells
✘ Sour cream
✘ Guacamole
✘ Shredded (higher-fat) cheese
✘ Mexican cheese or sausage (chorizo)
✘ Chimichangas
✘ Crispy, deep-fried foods
✘ Refried beans

Ask your server to do this:

▶ Hold the sour cream, guacamole
▶ Remove the chips
▶ Serve salad without taco shell
▶ Hold the cheese
▶ Put on some extra shredded lettuce and tomatoes

## Pizza

Pizza is a mainstay in the American diet. Not only can you find the old standby of thin crust with cheese, but you are able to order almost any type of stuffed crust and pizza stuffed with anything and everything imaginable. Be careful with your pizza selections. They can provide a wide variety of healthier vegetables to your diet or be a high-fat, high-calorie nutrition disaster.

Healthier options include the following.

✔ Thin crust
✔ Green and red peppers
✔ Mushrooms
✔ Onions
✔ Tomatoes
✔ Broccoli
✔ Eggplant
✔ Garlic
✔ Spinach
✔ Chicken, shrimp
✔ Artichoke hearts
✔ Canadian bacon
✔ Low-fat cheese

Be cautious of these things:

✘ Extra cheese
✘ Stuffed crusts and stuffed pizzas
✘ Pepperoni
✘ Sausage
✘ Anchovies
✘ Bacon
✘ Ground meat
✘ Prosciutto
✘ Olives

Ask the server to do this:

▶ Start you off with a side salad, low-fat dressing on the side
▶ Substitute low-fat cheese
▶ Top with lots of extra vegetables
▶ Go light on the cheese

# Packing Lunches to Go

Many people do find it necessary to pack lunches. Whether for work, school, or at the ball field, packing a lunch can be a healthy option for many people. Carrying a lunch does offer you nutrition benefits over fast-food choices or the vending machine. When you pack your own lunch, you know what goes into it. Of course, you can also save money as well.

Packing lunch while keeping nutrition guidelines in mind is the best way to focus on a healthier meal away from home. A well-balanced lunch should contain a high-protein food, a starch, a fruit and/or vegetable, and a beverage. Occasionally a treat could be thrown in too. When packing your lunch, try to look back at the Food Guide Pyramid for healthy suggestions. Choose foods from each of the food groups. Limit excess snack foods, cookies, candies, and cakes that are high in fat and sugar. Select high-fiber foods, too, like whole-grain breads and rolls and fresh fruits and vegetable sticks.

**ALERT**

When packing lunches, keep food safety in mind. If your lunch will not be refrigerated, use appropriate containers to keep them at proper temperatures. You can freeze a juice box or use an ice pack to keep them cool.

Sandwiches typically are the number one choice for many packed lunches. Seek out new fillings and new types of breads and rolls to make your sandwich more appealing. How about some sliced chicken or tuna? Or what about trying a focaccia roll or raisin bread? You can even try a thermos of soup, cottage cheese, or yogurt for a change. And don't forget about pasta salad. Leftovers from home also make good lunches, too.

Packing a good lunch does not take a lot of time. But it does take planning. If you find your mornings rushed, then pack your lunch the night before. When cleaning up leftovers, pack some into individual servings. These are often welcome choices for the next day's lunch. Seek out appropriate containers, too. These containers can help separate foods, insulate foods, and keep them fresh.

Just because you are watching your weight doesn't mean you cannot enjoy the pleasures of eating out. Whether you choose a full-service or fast-food restaurant, you need to make a conscious effort to plan and make wise food selections. As you become more knowledgeable as to what and how you should be eating, you will be able to eat out without a great deal of effort. Restaurants are also trying to cater to consumers' requests and needs. Many more choices are becoming available to us. As time goes on this will allow people everywhere to better meet their needs and desires while enjoying the benefits of eating out.

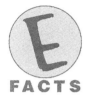

**FACTS**

A healthy lunch should consist of a high-protein food (such as sliced turkey, roast beef, yogurt, or hard-boiled egg), fresh fruit or vegetable (carrot sticks, cucumber slices, fresh peppers, grapes, or apple), bread or starch (bagel, whole-grain bread, crackers), a treat (fig bar, vanilla wafers, gingersnaps) and finally juice, water, or milk.

## CHAPTER 16

# Meal Planning and Shopping

lanning meals is just that—planning. Guidelines for planning meals and snacks are not set in stone and can be modified to fit into busy schedules, appointments, and lifestyles. But it is important to establish a system that works for you in order to manage your meals and snacks to the best of your abilities.

# Planning Appealing Meals

Have you ever served a meal that just did not look very appetizing to you? Let's say you're sitting down to a meal of baked chicken, mashed potatoes, and cauliflower on a white dinner plate, or maybe a fresh stir-fry with a side salad. Did your chicken meal look too white in color and very bland on the plate? Or when you ate your stir-fry dinner, did you feel like everything you ate was too crunchy? Meals like these often happen when we do not plan what will be served.

**E**SSENTIALS
To easily plan your meals, do so on a cycle menu: Monday (chicken), Tuesday (fish), Wednesday (vegetarian), Thursday (beef), Friday (pasta), Saturday (leftovers), Sunday (ethnic). Make a chart, starting with your favorite main-dish recipe, and add complementary side dishes.

A meal should be appealing. If it is not, it will not be enjoyed. A proper meal should be one that is rich in color, flavor, texture, and nutrients.

## Color

The color of your meal appeals to your eye and starts to stimulate your appetite when you see it. If the meal is all one color, it doesn't look nearly as appealing as one that presents a collection of various colors. Remember the meal described above—this all-white plate can be made more appealing by changing it to baked chicken with wild rice and fresh broccoli spears. Doesn't that sound better to you?

## Flavor

Flavor is an important component of meals as well. Sometimes spicy is appetizing, other times a sweeter touch may be in order. Again, keep in mind that the variety of foods presented should carry different flavors. All spicy or all sweet foods may be too much at one time. Try offering some mild beans or rice with a spicy enchilada, rather than a spicy side dish, to help balance your taste buds. The temperature of your meal should also be considered. Most people enjoy a balance of some hot foods with cold foods. Soup and fresh salad go well together, as does an omelet with fresh orange juice.

## Texture

The texture of foods should also be thought out in advance. People like the combination of soft foods with crunchy or chewy foods. Eating a meal should be a pleasant experience, not one that requires an excessive amount of chewing or no chewing at all.

## Nutrients

And finally, a meal should be full of a wide range of nutrients. It is easier to put together a nutritious meal by choosing foods from the different food groups and planning a range of colorful food selections and various flavors and textures. Fiber is abundant in fresh, crunchy foods. Vitamins A and C can be found in both dark green leafy and red vegetables. Protein is abundant in meats, and calcium is found in dairy sources. Following suggestions of foods provided in the Food Guide Pyramid (Chapter 6) you will be able to plan meals that provide recommended daily nutrients. The food pyramid also helps you control the fat, cholesterol, sugar, and sodium in your meals while including the rich sources of vitamins, minerals, fiber, and other important nutrients.

# Managing Your Food Budget

Busy schedules often dictate when many people do their grocery shopping. Often, mom may stop at the store between carpooling to pick up a few items for dinner, or dad stops by the store on his way home from work. In any case, when a few items are picked up here and there, more money is spent in the long run. These quick trips to the grocery store also allure shoppers to buy tempting foods placed inside the front door or those they may not necessarily need.

To get the most from your dollar, try some of the following tricks.

- Plan your meals.

- Keep a shopping list.
- Avoid grocery shopping when you are hungry, tired, or in a hurry.
- Buy store specials and foods in season.
- Keep coupons for items you typically buy.
- Stock your pantry and refrigerator with staples.
- Buy package sizes that you know you will use; don't buy large sizes just because they are cheaper if you know you will not use all the food.
- Comparison shop; read unit price shelf labels and the Nutrition Facts labels.

## Shopping Within Your Needs

Shopping on your family's food budget requires planning in itself. Your budget will help you to properly plan to balance your income to fit the needs of your expenses. If you are responsible for your family's food shopping, it would be wise for you to estimate your food needs and aim to stay within that budget. Buying foods in season, clipping coupons, and watching store specials help in keeping food expenses under control. Planning to shop once each week, stocking the pantry and refrigerator properly, and limiting those quick stops at the convenience store helps keep your food budget from getting out of hand.

**ALERT**

Look up and down as you walk down the aisles. The more expensive name-brand items are usually placed at eye level. Generic and bargain-brands are set up on higher or down on lower shelves, and they require more effort to locate them.

## Comparison Shopping

It is also in your best interest to learn to comparison shop. This means to compare two or more similar products to determine the one that best meets your needs and budget. Many grocery stores offer shelf labels to indicate unit prices. This means they have done some comparison shopping for you. Here, the labels tell consumers how much the food item costs per standard unit of weight or volume. In other words, the label tells you how much a box of name-brand dry cereal may cost per ounce as compared to a box of similarly packaged generic cereal. By reading these shelf labels, you can decide for yourself which package is best suited to your needs.

**FIGURE 16-1:**
Comparison
of shelf labels

**6 oz.**
**NAME BRAND**
**CHUNK LIGHT TUNA**

**$1.29**
**.21 per**
**ounce**

**6 oz.**
**GENERIC BRAND**
**CHUNK LIGHT TUNA**

**$.89**
**.14 per**
**ounce**

- Look for unit price (the cost per standard unit of weight or volume).
- Determine which product best suits your needs.
- Look to save money on comparible items when the less expensive (most likely the store brand or generic item) item will work for you.

## Preparing Shopping Lists

One of the best ways to plan for the food items you need is to create a standard shopping list. Keeping this list handy at home helps family members to keep up-to-date on foods that need to be purchased. Take this list with you to the store and stick with it; it will keep you on target as to what you need. Otherwise, impulse shopping can cause you to buy many products you may not have planned to buy.

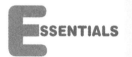

**E**SSENTIALS

When time is limited, convenience items can be a good choice. But be wise when making your selections. And add complementary lower-fat side dishes to accompany higher-fat main dishes.

Try this sample shopping list for your needs.

## Shopping List

### Fresh Fruits and Vegetables

| | | |
|---|---|---|
| _____ | _____ | _____ |
| _____ | _____ | _____ |
| _____ | _____ | _____ |

### Fresh Meats/Poultry/Fish

☐ Chicken   ☐ Beef   ☐ Pork   ☐ Fish   ☐ Other

| | | |
|---|---|---|
| _____ | _____ | _____ |
| _____ | _____ | _____ |
| _____ | _____ | _____ |

### Dairy/Refrigerated Foods

☐ Milk   ☐ Eggs   ☐ Margarine

☐ Cheese   ☐ Yogurt

| | | |
|---|---|---|
| _____ | _____ | _____ |
| _____ | _____ | _____ |
| _____ | _____ | _____ |

## Grain Products

☐ Bread ☐ Bagels ☐ English muffins

☐ Pasta ☐ Cereal ☐ Rice

_____  _____  _____
_____  _____  _____
_____  _____  _____

## Convenience Snack Foods/Packaged Foods

☐ Crackers ☐ Fruit/Granola bars ☐ Pretzels ☐ Popcorn

_____  _____  _____
_____  _____  _____
_____  _____  _____

## Canned/Jar Foods

☐ Pasta sauce ☐ Tomato Sauce/Paste

☐ Soup/Broths ☐ Fruits/Vegetables

_____  _____  _____
_____  _____  _____
_____  _____  _____

## Other Foods and Condiments

_____  _____  _____
_____  _____  _____
_____  _____  _____

Do I have coupons? ☐ Yes ☐ No

## Store specials to check

_____  _____  _____
_____  _____  _____
_____  _____  _____

# Prepackaged/Convenience Foods

Prepackaged and convenience foods show up regularly on shopping lists and in shopping carts. These foods can save time and energy when preparing meals, but they can also run up your food bill rather quickly. Estimate the cost of preparing certain foods from scratch, and then compare them to the prepackaged item. See what the difference is for you? Making these foods from scratch can also save you additional calories and fat, as many of these convenience items offer many more calories and fat than you may add to your home-cooked product. Making fried rice from a prepared rice mix is much more caloric than a quick, home-prepared version If you are a fan of macaroni and cheese, you may find you can use lower-fat cheese and milk when you prepare it yourself, an option that may not be available in a prepackaged type.

**ESSENTIALS** Health claims must meet standard criteria and can be made through statements, symbols (like a heart), or descriptions.

Also, watch those frozen dinners. Many weight-conscious consumers opt to purchase the frozen meals available today. There are entrées, family-size varieties, side dishes, and even special meals catering to children. Sometimes these meals are a good choice for consumers in that they offer standard serving sizes and sometimes use lower-fat preparation methods. Some of these meals also offer vegetables and fruits that many people neglect in their homemade meals.

When selecting frozen meals, aim to meet these guidelines:

- Select meals with no more than 30 percent of total calories from fat.
- Select meals with no more than 200 milligrams of sodium per 100 calories.
- Select meals with at least 40 percent of the Recommended Dietary Allowances for vitamins A and C.

Keep in mind that these guidelines don't guarantee that daily recommendations are being met for each and every nutrient. In order to ensure a healthy intake, consumers need to alternate their food choices, limit everyday consumption of frozen meals, and learn to compensate for missing nutrients during other meals and snacks during the day.

# Stock Those Staples

A very important component of eating healthy and losing weight is shopping for healthy foods and stocking a home full of good food choices. Shopping at least once each week, with a list in hand, helps keep a good variety of perishable and lower-fat fresh foods available. This allows you to always have a variety of foods available for quick and healthy meals and snacks.

## Learning the Layout of Your Supermarket

When you shop, try to do so at the same supermarket each week. Get to know the layout and the location of various foods. Supermarkets are designed to tempt you to buy more food than you may normally. Did you ever wonder why the milk and meat counters are always the farthest from the front door? Or why stores are now baking bread in the afternoons? Milk and meat are the two most purchased items in the grocery store. When you run in to grab a gallon of milk and have to walk up and down various aisles, you will be more tempted to pick up one or two additional items. And those delicious baked breads smell so tempting on a quick stop at the store after work. Marketers plan for these to appeal to you. Haven't you ever run into the store for one item and come out with ten? It happens all the time.

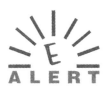

**ALERT**

Shop the outer perimeter of your store for the freshest and most nutritious food choices.

Your best bet when shopping is to begin at the store's perimeter. The outer aisles are stocked with most of your staples. The inside aisles mainly stock processed, convenience-type foods. Fruits and vegetables, fresh meats and seafood, dairy products, and fresh breads are usually found along the walls of the store, while dry cereals, canned goods, pasta and sauces, cookies, crackers, beverages, and soups are often in inner aisles. Use your shopping list and try to stick with it for the best selection of food items.

## Guide to Stocking Your Home

Here are some recommendations to help you stock your home with healthful food choices:

- Whole-grain breads
- Bagels
- Pita bread
- English muffins
- Rye or pumpernickel breads
- Raisin bread
- Assorted sugar-free dry cereals
- Oatmeal
- Brown rice
- Couscous
- Bread crumbs
- Pasta
- Low-fat frozen waffles and pancakes
- Skinless, boneless chicken breasts
- Lean ground beef or turkey
- Lean cuts of beef (flank, sirloin, tenderloin)
- Lean cuts of pork (canned, cured, boiled ham; Canadian bacon; pork tenderloin)
- Fresh fish (white fish, turbot, fillet of sole, salmon), frozen fish without breading
- Tuna, sardines, packed in water
- Skim or low-fat milk

- Eggs
- Low-fat ricotta cheese
- Low-fat cottage cheese or sliced cheese
- Nonfat or low-fat yogurts
- Nonfat or low-fat sour cream
- Margarine or diet spreads
- Parmesan cheese
- Low-fat granola or fruit bars
- Low-fat or fat-free cookies (vanilla wafers, gingersnaps)
- Fruit-filled cookie bars
- Low-fat crackers
- Baked tortilla chips
- Pretzels
- Popcorn (low-fat microwave popcorn)
- Rice cakes
- Cantaloupe/honeydew melons
- Apples
- Bananas
- Kiwi fruit
- Grapes
- Oranges/grapefruit
- Raspberries/blueberries/strawberries
- Pineapple
- Lemons
- Plums/nectarines
- Raisins/dried fruits
- Canned fruit (juice packed)
- Applesauce
- 100 percent fruit juices
- Carrots, baby carrots
- Cauliflower
- Celery
- Cucumbers
- Cabbage, napa cabbage
- Onions

- Broccoli
- Zucchini
- White or sweet potatoes
- Peppers (green, red, yellow)
- Lettuce, romaine, bibb, spinach, or other varieties
- Tomatoes
- Frozen vegetables (without sauce)
- Canned tomatoes
- Tomato sauces, paste
- Canned beans
- Pasta sauces
- Pizza crusts
- Vegetarian burgers
- Low-fat soups
- Chicken/beef/vegetable broths
- Salsa
- Light mayonnaise
- Lemon juice
- Cooking sprays
- Balsamic/red wine vinegar
- Oils, vegetable and olive
- Mustard
- Light soy sauce
- Low-fat salad dressings
- Light syrups/fruit spreads
- Spices and herbs of choice

**ESSENTIALS** Every home should be stocked with a variety of food staples. Use your discretion on those that serve you best.

You do not need to purchase all these foods at once, but it is a good idea to try to keep many of them on hand. Having this selection available will allow you to prepare many quick and healthy meals without a great deal of time and thought. As you begin to properly stock your home of appropriate types of foods, you will notice how beneficial they really are. Our staple selections can eventually become your staple favorites. You may also wish to remove items in your home that no longer fit your eating style, or any food that has been sitting in your home for extended lengths of time. Clean out items like candies, cookies, snack foods, and presweetened cereals and begin to enjoy the fresh, delicious taste of wholesome, nutritious food instead.

# Reading Food Labels

Nutrition Facts labels found on food products are your primary source of information about what nutrients are found in the various foods. Food labeling guidelines are regulated by the U.S. Food and Drug Administration, while the U.S. Department of Agriculture governs the labels found on meat and poultry products. Federal laws do require foods to carry Nutrition Facts labels on every product that is processed or packaged.

ALERT

If you haven't used a particular food in over a year, get rid of it. You will likely not use it (or want to use it) in the future.

Manufacturers' name and addresses, along with the food distribution company, must also appear, along with a nutrition panel that provides a listing of ingredients and standard nutrients.

## Ingredient List

Federal law requires that all food ingredients be listed on the label. These ingredients, listed in descending order by weight, include all substances found in the food. This information is important for people who need to avoid certain types of foods in their diet due to special dietary needs, religious reasons, or because of a food intolerance or allergy.

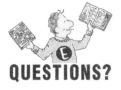

**Are there any food products that are exempt from federal food labeling laws?**

Yes, complete nutrition labels are not necessary for foods prepared by small businesses, bakeries, and restaurants. Food in multiunit packages, those in small packages like chewing gum, and coffee and tea are also exempt.

## Health and Nutrient Claims

You have seen product labels that say "reduced fat," "low cholesterol," or "sugar free." Or how about a claim about the benefits of calcium in preventing the risk of osteoporosis or reducing fat to prevent certain types of cancers? Health and nutrient claims are often found on food labels. As a matter of fact, these claims are placed on the labels to sway a consumer to purchase one particular item over another one. Manufacturers include these claims to help sell their product. In some cases these products may be a better choice, other times not. Just because a label indicates that the product is "light" doesn't always mean it is a lower in fat or calories; it could also be lighter in color or in sodium. Be a smart consumer and learn to compare one product against another to determine if one has greater value over another before you buy.

The good news is that the federal government regulates these claims. Health claims are based on scientific research showing evidence of the connection between foods or nutrients and specific diseases. Statements listed can indicate that a specific diet/health relationship exists, but statements cannot indicate that a certain food or food product prevents or causes a disease.

The following health claims are the only ones currently permitted to be printed on food labels:

- **Calcium and Osteoporosis:** A calcium-rich diet is linked to a reduced risk of osteoporosis, a condition in which bones become soft or brittle.
- **Fat and cancer:** A diet low in total fat is linked to a reduced risk of some cancers.

- **Saturated fat and cholesterol and heart disease:** A diet low in saturated fat and cholesterol can help reduce the risk of heart disease.
- **Fiber-containing grain products, fruits, and vegetables, and cancer:** A diet rich in high-fiber grain products, fruits, and vegetables can reduce the risk of some cancers.
- **Fruits, vegetables, and grain products that contain fiber and risk of heart disease:** A diet rich in fruits, vegetables, and grain products that contain fiber can help reduce the risk for heart disease.
- **Sodium and high blood pressure (hypertension):** A low-sodium diet may help reduce the risk of high blood pressure, which is a risk factor for heart attacks and strokes.
- **Fruits and vegetables and cancer:** A low-fat diet rich in fruits and vegetables (foods that are low in fat and may contain dietary fiber, vitamin A, or vitamin C) is linked to a reduced risk of some cancers.
- **Folic acid and neural tube defects:** Women who consume .4 milligrams of folic acid per day reduce their risk of giving birth to a child affected with a neural tube defect.

Nutrient content claims are more specific than health claims. In order for a product to include any of these claims, the food product must meet appropriate criteria.

| THIS CLAIM . . . | IS DEFINED AS . . . |
|---|---|
| Calorie free | fewer than 5 calories per serving |
| Low calorie | 40 calories or fewer per serving |
| Reduced (fewer) calories | at least 25 percent fewer calories per serving than the regular version |
| Light or lite | a third fewer calories or 50 percent less fat or less sodium per serving than the regular version |
| Sugar free | fewer than .5 grams of sugar per serving |
| Reduced sugar or less sugar | at least 25 percent less sugar per serving |
| No added sugar | no sugars added during processing or packing, including ingredients that contain sugars, such as juice or dried fruit |

| THIS CLAIM . . . | IS DEFINED AS . . . |
| --- | --- |
| Fat free | fewer than .5 grams of fat per serving |
| Low fat | 3 grams or fewer of fat per serving |
| Reduced (less) fat | at least 25 percent less fat per serving |
| Lean (meats) | fewer than 10 grams of fat per serving, and 4.5 grams or less of saturated fat, and 95 milligrams of cholesterol per serving |
| Extra lean (meats) | fewer than 5 grams of fat per serving and less than 2 grams of saturated fat and 95 milligrams of cholesterol per serving |
| Cholesterol free | fewer than 2 milligrams of cholesterol and 2 grams or less of saturated fat per serving |
| Low cholesterol | 20 milligrams or fewer of cholesterol and 2 grams or less of saturated fat per serving |
| Reduced (less) cholesterol | at least 25 percent less cholesterol and 2 grams or less of saturated fat per serving |
| Sodium free | fewer than 5 milligrams of sodium per serving |
| Very low sodium | 35 milligrams or fewer of sodium per serving |
| Low sodium | 140 milligrams or fewer of sodium per serving |
| Reduced (less) sodium | at least 25 percent less sodium per serving |

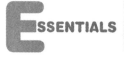

**ESSENTIALS**   In food labels, total fat and calories provide the most commonly used information for individuals watching their weight.

## The Nutrition Facts Label

The most informative part of the food label is found within the Nutrition Facts panel. Here information is provided about the food product on a per serving basis. The panel indicates the recommended serving size, number of calories in a serving, the number of calories from fat in a serving, and amounts of nutrients per serving, including total fat, saturated fat, cholesterol, sodium, total carbohydrates, dietary fiber, sugars, and protein. Amounts for these nutrients are listed in grams or milligrams per serving as well as in percentage of Daily Values. Daily Values are also required to be included for vitamins A and C, calcium, and iron.

As illustrated in **FIGURE 16-2**, the Nutrition Facts panel offers much information to help consumers make good choices about the foods they eat. Individuals seeking to lose weight and modify caloric intake can use this information to purchase foods that help limit their fat intake to 30 percent or less of total calories.

The bottom of the Nutrition Facts panel offers reference information for consumers on daily intake limits of fat, saturated fat, cholesterol, and sodium, and appropriate intake for total carbohydrate and dietary fiber for both a 2,000- and 2,500-calorie diet. This information assists in helping consumers see how a particular product fits into a total day's requirement.

**FIGURE 16-2:**
Nutrition
Facts panel

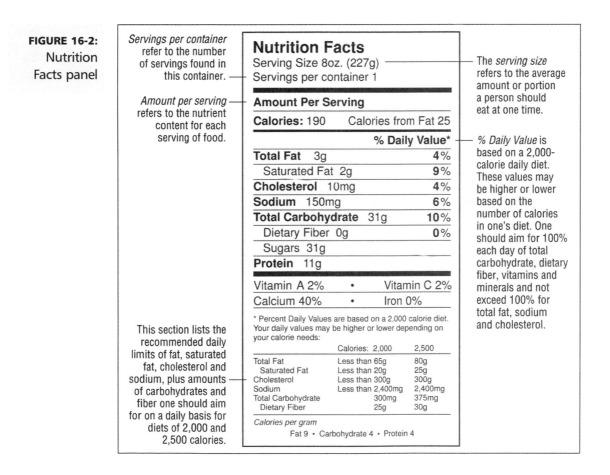

*Servings per container* refer to the number of servings found in this container.

*Amount per serving* refers to the nutrient content for each serving of food.

This section lists the recommended daily limits of fat, saturated fat, cholesterol and sodium, plus amounts of carbohydrates and fiber one should aim for on a daily basis for diets of 2,000 and 2,500 calories.

The *serving size* refers to the average amount or portion a person should eat at one time.

*% Daily Value* is based on a 2,000-calorie daily diet. These values may be higher or lower based on the number of calories in one's diet. One should aim for 100% each day of total carbohydrate, dietary fiber, vitamins and minerals and not exceed 100% for total fat, sodium and cholesterol.

## Nutrition Facts
Serving Size 8oz. (227g)
Servings per container 1

**Amount Per Serving**

**Calories:** 190          Calories from Fat 25

|  | **% Daily Value*** |
|---|---|
| **Total Fat**   3g | **4**% |
| Saturated Fat  2g | **9**% |
| **Cholesterol**   10mg | **4**% |
| **Sodium**   150mg | **6**% |
| **Total Carbohydrate**   31g | **10**% |
| Dietary Fiber  0g | **0**% |
| Sugars  31g | |
| **Protein**   11g | |

| | | | |
|---|---|---|---|
| Vitamin A 2% | • | Vitamin C 2% |
| Calcium 40% | • | Iron 0% |

\* Percent Daily Values are based on a 2,000 calorie diet. Your daily values may be higher or lower depending on your calorie needs:

|  | Calories: | 2,000 | 2,500 |
|---|---|---|---|
| Total Fat | Less than | 65g | 80g |
| Saturated Fat | Less than | 20g | 25g |
| Cholesterol | Less than | 300g | 300g |
| Sodium | Less than | 2,400mg | 2,400mg |
| Total Carbohydrate | | 300mg | 375mg |
| Dietary Fiber | | 25g | 30g |

*Calories per gram*
Fat 9 • Carbohydrate 4 • Protein 4

Total fat recommendations are based on 30 percent of total calorie needs for the day. To determine your specific needs if you are not following a 2,000- or 2,500-calorie diet, you need to divide your total calories by .30 (30 percent). For example, if you are following a 1,500-calorie diet, no more than 450 daily calories should come from fat (1,500 × .30 = 450). To change this to grams of fat, you divide 450 by 9. (Fat provides 9 calories per gram of food.) Therefore, you should aim for a maximum of 50 grams of fat per day. (You can also refer to the chart in Chapter 5 for further details.)

Keep the following tips in mind when reading food labels:

- Stick with listed serving size. Consuming more than this amount leads to higher calories consumed.
- Watch package sizes. Some products such as beverages, prepackaged foods, and tuna may look like one serving, but they are actually two. Refer to the "servings per container" reference on the label for complete and accurate guidance.
- Look for high-fiber foods with at least 5 grams of dietary fiber per serving. These foods help fill you up and are often lower in fat and calories than others.
- Watch calories from fat. Make sure you are not consuming too much fat as your primary nutrient source.
- Balance your food choices. For every higher-fat product you choose, balance your meal with a lower-fat option. For example, balance cheese cubes with rice cakes or whole wheat crackers.

Eating healthy, and losing weight as a result, isn't all about eating. It encompasses much more, as you have read in this chapter. Planning, shopping, and reading and understanding nutrition labels are all a part of successful weight management and creating healthier eating habits. No one can just change their eating habits overnight. Change takes time and change requires planning. Take it slow, and as you do your habits will change for the better and change for good.

## CHAPTER 17

# Taking It off and Keeping It Off

L osing and maintaining weight loss isn't just about cutting out calories, reducing overall food intake, or following an exercise program. Losing weight and keeping it off permanently is a lifelong process, not something that can occur quickly and soon be forgotten. As much as each of us would like to make temporary changes and see results overnight, this is not realistic.

## Accepting Body Weight

First and foremost, get past your obsession with body weight. Body weight should not be your number one concern—body composition and health should be.

Weight gain is inevitable as we age. Our metabolism decreases throughout our adult lives, somewhere in the area of 3 to 5 percent each decade. It is not unusual for men and women who have not had any weight issues their entire life to put on an additional 10 to 15 pounds during their adult years. That amount of additional weight is manageable. Those additional pounds should not add any major health risks. But we do need to be concerned when weight increases to levels of 20 pounds or more, especially if those pounds are in areas surrounding our body's vital organs. When this occurs, health risks and risk of diseases are increased and even premature deaths can occur.

The bathroom scale should not be your sole guide to your weight concerns. Put the bathroom scale away, or at least keep it out of sight on a daily basis. Staying focused on a number on the bathroom scale can wreak havoc with your attitude. The number on the scale does not reflect on you as a person. Body weight fluctuates daily due to water weight and monthly cycles in women. Focus on health, not weight. If you do feel compelled to check in with your bathroom scale, do so on a weekly or monthly basis, at the same time of day, without clothing, and on the same scale.

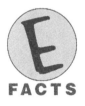

**FACTS**

Losing weight and maintaining a healthy weight requires much more than just cutting calories. It involves a lifelong approach to healthy eating and incorporation of positive lifestyle habits.

Accept yourself for who you are. Not everyone is tall or short. Nor is everyone thin and trim. If you have had a problem with weight your entire life, it may be difficult to make a total change to your body in adulthood. Just aim to be the best and healthiest person you can be. Learn to feel good about who you are, what you can do for yourself, and how you make others feel around you. Do the best you can, and be the best you can be.

# Setting Realistic Goals

Make realistic and reasonable goals for yourself. It is great to set goals for yourself both for the short and the long term. Losing weight and being healthier and more fit is important, but those goals should not get in the way of enjoying your life. People often seek unrealistic targets rather than doing the best they can for themselves. This can set them up for failure. Instead of focusing on "I want to lose 20 pounds before my high school reunion next month" strive for "I will walk two miles each day to feel better overall." The short-term goals can ultimately help you to accomplish those long-term results.

**E**SSENTIALS

Body weight is not as important as body composition. The scale should not be your number one indicator of your health.

Use a weekly calendar or your personal dietary diary to jot down your goals. First, identify problem areas in your eating, exercise, and behavior patterns. Then note the changes you can make to your current habits. When you write them down, these goals become a constant reminder for you to follow. Make a commitment with yourself to stick with your goals. Take it one step and one day at a time. Soon enough results will follow. Don't forget to evaluate your goals frequently, maybe once each week, to see how you are doing. Reward yourself (not with food, of course). Once you have mastered one goal, move on to another. This will keep you motivated over the long haul.

# Creating Meal Plans

Focus on a healthy diet, not a restrictive one. Create a meal plan that works for you. Incorporate meals and snacks that fit into your schedule. Whether you are a single person with a busy job or a parent of active toddlers, an appropriate plan that includes regular meals and snacks should be made.

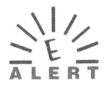

Carrying extra body weight around the middle of one's body is more critical than carrying excess weight around the hips, thighs, and buttocks. Too much weight surrounding the body's vital organs can lead to additional risk of illness and disease.

## Balance, Variety, and Moderation

Here again, I want to reiterate the importance of balance, variety, and moderation in everything you do. The foods you eat, the activities you choose, and the lifestyle you lead all should include a balanced selection, a variety of good choices, and moderation.

Balancing your food groups, selecting variety within each food group, and consuming foods within moderation are all key to healthy eating and to losing and maintaining healthy weight effectively. You can also think of these words in terms of daily activity. Balancing your body's activities, selecting a variety of fitness and sports options, and practicing them within moderation will help keep you fit, too.

Eating a healthy, well-balanced selection of foods that incorporates a variety of food choices in moderate portions is your key to healthy eating. Choose high-complex carbohydrates that include whole grains, fruits, and vegetables, along with many lower-fat foods to balance choices found in the Food Guide Pyramid. This new way of looking at your food intake will benefit in helping you enjoy your foods without feeling deprived.

Focus on your overall food intake, not just the "good foods" and "bad foods." All foods can fit into your diet, in moderation.

Enjoy an occasional treat along with other food choices. Don't deprive yourself as you can then set yourself up for failure. Forbidden foods become that much more desirable.

And again, keep track of your food choices in your diet diary. Log them by individual food item and based on which food group they fall into. By doing so, you are educating yourself on how and what you should be eating. Each step brings you closer to a happier and healthier you.

## Watch Those Portion Sizes

Portion control is key. Moderation is so important when choosing and making food selections. All foods can fit into any lifestyle. It's the amount that must be watched. Fast foods, buffet items, desserts, alcoholic beverages, and the like can really add up. Be cautious of higher-fat and higher-calorie foods, and opt for more selections that are lower in fat, lower in calories, and higher in fiber.

**FACTS**

Not every person can be thin and trim, but every person can be healthy.

Stay clear of second servings, spoonfuls at the stove, or handfuls of treats here and there. Each and every bite adds up, whether it's eaten at the table, out of the refrigerator, in the car, or at the sampling counter at the supermarket.

## Don't Forget the Fiber

Push the fiber. Fiber helps provide the sensation of feeling full. People who eat high-fiber diets tend to eat less food overall. Fiber can also prevent digestive problems associated with constipation and diverticulitis.

Opt for whole grains, fruits and vegetables, and beans and legumes to increase your fiber intake. Not only are these foods high in fiber, but they are low in calories and fat, too.

## Create a Plan that Works for You

Plan your meals and snacks, and write the plan down. Good eating and good habits require planning. Find out what process works best for you. Try setting up a cycle menu to give yourself of the types of foods you want to serve on any particular day of the week. Plan side dishes as well as main courses. And don't forget variety in color, flavors, and textures.

Keep an ongoing shopping list on your refrigerator. Here, you will notice when you have run out of foods and staples and you will be able to keep good choices on hand. Also stock your pantry, freezer, and refrigerator properly. If you have a wide variety of foods available, you will most likely use them. And the contrary is true, too. If only poor choices are available, these will be the foods consumed.

## Keeping Active

Keep as active as you can be. The American public weighs more today than it ever has before, mainly due to increased sedentary lifestyles. Physical activity is a key factor in weight loss and weight management.

Find activities you enjoy. Walking . . . biking . . . skating . . . running . . . dancing. A combination of strength training and aerobic conditioning can help exercise your heart while helping you to lose fat. Almost every person who succeeds at weight loss does so through increased physical activity. Exercise makes you feel good about yourself. People who exercise regularly generally are happier and have less stress, too.

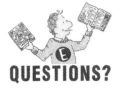

**QUESTIONS?**

**What exactly is a weight-loss plateau?**
A weight-loss plateau is a state during which your body temporarily resists losing weight. Sometimes this is a result of water retention. Other times this is just a means to get your body adjusted to a different weight. Keep with your program. Eventually you will see results again.

Again, keep track of what you do. Make a list of activities you would like to try and others you do regularly. Enlist friends to join you and motivate you. Make activity a priority for first thing in the morning, if necessary. You will feel much better for your accomplishments later in the day.

## Making Changes to Last a Lifetime

Make gradual lifestyle changes. You didn't create your old habits overnight, and you shouldn't expect to create new habits that quickly either. Making small changes will add up to big results. If it takes you months or a year to create new habits, work on them slowly. Each and every change can be beneficial in the long run.

**FACTS**

There are no "good foods" and no "bad foods," only "good diets" and "bad diets."

Obviously we have learned that the most effective weight-loss program is based on changing lifestyle habits. That includes eating healthfully, exercising regularly, and maintaining other healthy habits, such as avoiding smoking and limiting alcohol consumption. Habits that led to problems with overweight and obesity now need to be replaced with habits that lead to health and fitness goals.

## Small Changes Add Up

Eating to lose and maintain weight, increasing activity, and changing inappropriate behaviors aren't just the result of a one-time overhaul but of small practical and realistic changes to one's lifestyle. Take one day at a time and make one change at a time. Initially you may want to try eating more slowly, eating only at the kitchen table, and serving meals at the stove rather than on the table to avoid grabbing second servings.

Additional changes could include cutting back on an afternoon snack twice a week, or not eating after 9:00 P.M., or even walking around the block once a day. Once you make the change, move on to another. Remember small changes add up to big results. Do whatever works best for you.

## Moving Past Plateaus

Anticipate ups and down. Gradual changes to your lifestyle will add changes to your overall weight, but don't expect miracles. Your body has to adjust to changes and will fight you along the way. You may initially lose some water weight, thus increasing your motivation to continue, but weight does stabilize and you will notice some plateaus. Just keep it up and positive results will continue.

Plateaus are common occurrences in long-term weight reduction. Dieters often get discouraged and frustrated when the weight loss stops. As you continue to lose weight your body begins to adjust to its new weight. By doing so it becomes accustomed to meeting energy needs for a lesser weight. Losing weight becomes more and more difficult as you approach your weight goal. But it isn't impossible to get there. It just takes a little more effort. Don't view these plateaus as a failure but as a time to jump-start your plan.

To jump-start your weight-loss plan to avoid plateaus, follow these tips:

- **Redefine your goals:** Address those areas that are most important to you now.
- **Evaluate your food intake:** You may be consuming more than you realize.
- **Boost your exercise routine:** Find ways to boost your metabolism; add an extra five to ten minutes each day, increase your intensity, and challenge yourself more.
- **Be consistent with keeping your diet and exercise diary:** Keeping accurate records will keep you on track.

## Accept Mistakes

Don't blame yourself if you make a mistake. We all make mistakes. Get past it and move on. Learn from your mistakes and attempt to make better choices the next time.

As you incorporate new changes into your lifestyle and aim to change your habits, you will slip back from time to time into old routines. Just learn to become aware of these relapses. By evaluating yourself on a continual basis, redefining goals, and planning ahead, you can stay on top of your concerns.

Whatever you do, don't get discouraged. Remember that you're just human! Don't let one relapse set you back. Get over it and move on. Learn from your mistakes. You will be happier in the long run.

# Resisting Fads and Trends

Each and every day, new fads and trends crack into the world of dieting. Whether they are magazine articles, pills, powders, beverages, or equipment, more and more efforts are made to lure the public into quick weight loss.

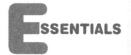

Engaging in a regular exercise routine, along with following a healthy, well-balanced diet, is the best way to maintain weight loss for life.

All sound tempting, but keep your good nutritional sense together. Don't be taken in with these claims. Yes, they are tempting, but no, they do not hold up for the long haul. You will soon be looking for the next fad or seeking alternatives once again in your future.

## Beware of the "Too Good to Be True" Promises

Don't be tempted by advertisement schemes. Any super promises, special formulas, fat-burning concoctions, and fat-loss creams are a waste of your hard-earned money. Don't be taken in by these promises. They simply do not work. Yes, you may lose some weight temporarily, but the loss is not permanent. And not the all-dreaded fat weight you long to lose. Often some of these products may actually cause more harm than good. These products also sidetrack you into trendy habits that cannot survive in the long term.

## Steer Clear of Severely Restrictive Diet Plans

Avoid restrictive weight-loss diets. When calories are limited to less than 1,200 calories (for women) and 1,500 (for men), it is less likely that all of the essential nutrients are being consumed. Don't deprive yourself of adequate nutrition for quick results that will likely backfire. Also avoid diets that restrict certain food groups altogether or promote food combining. These diets can lead to an obsession and preoccupation with food that can cause future problems.

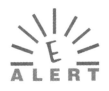

When you reduce food intake too much, your body will think you are trying to starve it. It will then protect itself by hanging on to all the fuel (food) it can get. As a result, your resting metabolism will decrease, thus making it more difficult to burn calories.

## Avoid Programs that Involve Fasting and Skipping Meals

Do not fast or skip meals. By doing so you will set yourself up for extreme hunger later in the day or in days to come.

When hunger strikes, all foods become tempting and you are likely to eat them in larger amounts. People who seek to lose weight often do better when they eat regularly, consume smaller meals, and sometimes eat up to six times during the course of a day. By doing so they continually feel full, avoid feeling extreme hunger, and learn to adjust to eating smaller portions more regularly throughout the day.

# Making the Transition from Losing to Maintaining

Once you achieve your weight goal, don't assume you are finished. Actually, you are just at a new beginning. You should be proud of your accomplishments. But unfortunately the weight maintenance can be more difficult than losing the weight in the first place.

Studies have demonstrated that a large percentage of people who lose weight actually gain it back within several months or up to a year after it is lost. Why? These individuals feel that they can resume their old habits once they reach their goal. They assume that they no longer need to watch their food intake, exercise as much, or continue to change their behaviors. But this is not the case at all. Each of these factors is key to maintaining the weight loss. Remember, this is a lifelong process, not a temporary change.

Once you reach your target weight goal, it is possible to eat more than before, but just a small amount more. To lose weight, you were reducing your intake about 500 calories per day. To maintain, you can add those calories back, but not more. These additional calories don't go a long way, so don't get carried away with them. These should be added from each of the food groups, not just treats, and in balanced proportions. Refer to the chart in Chapter 6 on recommended daily servings for maintaining health. This guide can help you incorporate additional servings into your daily meal plan to make up for those that were eliminated to allow for weight loss.

Should you opt for treats once in a while, be wise with your selections.

| NOT-SO-HEALTHY CHOICE | HEALTHY ALTERNATIVE |
| --- | --- |
| Potato chips | Air-popped popcorn, pretzels, low-fat crackers, fortified cereal, breadsticks, or low-fat chips |
| French fries | Baked potato, fresh fruit, no-fry french fries, or cut-up raw vegetables |
| Ice cream | Frozen yogurt, sherbet, sorbet, low-fat ice cream, or frozen fruit-pops |
| Soda pop | Unsweetened fruit juice with plain seltzer, iced tea, or ice water |
| Nachos with cheese | Plain tortilla chips or low-fat tortilla chips with bean, salsa, or low-fat dip |
| Donuts or pastries | Whole-grain cereal, whole-grain fruit bars, rice cakes, low-fat cookies, cookie bars, gingersnaps, or graham crackers |
| Candy bars | Low-fat granola bars, cereal bars, dried fruit, licorice, or hard candies |
| Rich deserts | Angel food cake with fruit topping, low-fat puddings, or sorbets |

Other great-tasting snacks under 100 calories include the following:

- 2 cups air-popped popcorn, unbuttered, sprinkled with Parmesan cheese
- 2 cups raw vegetables with low-fat dip
- $\frac{1}{3}$ cup whole-grain cereal
- 2 fig bars
- 1 piece or 1 cup fresh fruit
- 1 small apple with 1 tablespoon peanut butter
- 1 cup vegetarian vegetable soup
- $\frac{1}{2}$ cup sugar-free pudding made with skim milk
- $\frac{1}{2}$ pita bread filled with $\frac{1}{2}$ ounce low-fat shredded cheese
- 1 popsicle

Don't forget to go back and review your original goals. See if and when you accomplished each one, especially the long-term goals. If you have, set new ones. Just because you have met your weight-loss goals does not mean you should no longer strive to accomplish additional goals.

You should also take notice of changes. If you notice your clothes are beginning to tighten up a bit or feel you have put on a pound or two, take immediate action. Cut back again for a few days or a week to get back on track. It's a lot easier to lose 1 to 2 pounds than to take off 10 or 20. Be smart.

**QUESTIONS?**

**How can I avoid gaining my weight back?**
Initially, it is essential that you continue logging your food intake and exercise routines in a diet/exercise diary. As time goes by, you will become more comfortable with what you should and should not be doing. Remember the key words—balance, variety, and moderation.

There is never an end to eating right and exercising regularly. Every person, no matter how old, should have healthy habits throughout life. I know this isn't always the case, and that's I'm here to help you. If you have started off on the wrong foot, now is the time to make positive changes. Take action now, make the changes to eat better, lose the weight you want, and learn to maintain a happy, healthy lifestyle for the remainder of your years. Won't you be better off for it?

## CHAPTER 18

# Suggested Meal and Snack Plans

Some people enjoy the flexibility of making their own food choices and menu selections while other people like suggestions and ideas for putting together healthy, well-balanced meals. As you begin to make some changes in your lifestyle and food selections, you can choose to create your own meal plans or use some of these suggested plans.

## Evaluating Your Favorite Meals

As you first pull together your favorite recipes, see how many you can find. It's a fact that most people center their meals on the same twenty or so favorite meals and recipes over and over again while continuing to prepare and serve the same foods on a regular basis. Are you one of these people? Ask yourself to think (and list) the twenty most commonly prepared and served meals in your house.

Did you have difficulties coming up with twenty? Isn't it amazing how we feel like we spend so much time in the kitchen, collect so many recipes, have files and files of new ideas, and shelves of cookbooks, yet it is difficult to list twenty commonly prepared foods? This is not even enough to cover us for one month.

So take the time now to do something about it. First, throw away any recipes in your files that you have not prepared during the last year. Chances are that if you haven't made them recently, you probably won't be using them anytime soon. Next, start a new recipe file—in a drawer, shoebox, binder, or even on your personal computer. Finally, when you start to clip or save new recipes, try them first before you file them away. If they hold up to your satisfaction (and that of your family), file them appropriately. Then begin to incorporate them into your cycle menu or into weekly, or monthly, meal plans.

Later on in this book some of my favorite recipes are shared as well. Find some that appeal to you, and add them to your collection, too.

## Creating Meal Plans for Weight Loss

Back in Chapter 6, I gave recommendations as to the number of servings from each food group that should be incorporated into a daily diet. Suggestions included both recommendations for maintaining health and those for losing weight. Here, we will focus on those plans specifically designed for losing weight. The following meal plans meet these recommendations. You can choose to follow our sample plans or begin to create some of your own personalized plans, based on the same pattern.

To recap, here are the recommended daily servings for losing weight:

| FOOD GROUP | 1,200 CALORIES | 1,500 CALORIES | 1,800 CALORIES |
|---|---|---|---|
| Grain/Starch Group | 5 servings | 6 servings | 8 servings |
| Vegetable Group | 3 servings | 4 servings | 5 servings |
| Fruit Group | 2 servings | 3 servings | 4 servings |
| Dairy Group | 2 servings | 2 servings | 2 servings |
| Meat/Protein Group | 5 ounces | 6 ounces | 7 ounces |
| Fat/Oils/Sweets Group | limit to 1/day | limit to 1–2/day | limit to 2/day |

The following menu plans are based on the 1,500-calorie guidelines. If you prefer to follow those guidelines outlined in the 1,200- or 1,800-calorie levels, you will need to adjust your food groups servings accordingly. Keep in mind that these plans are provided to help with some ideas on how you can prepare and consume well-balanced, nutritious, lower-calorie meals. Balanced food choices incorporating a variety within each food group and in moderate portions remain the key to healthy low-fat meals. In order to maintain specific calorie levels, foods need to be prepared without excess fat and consumed in moderate portions.

## Using Meal Plans to Meet Your Needs

The following two-week collection of menu plans provides just a sampling of the types of meals you can prepare for yourself and your family. Each offers a wide variety of food choices, balances food groups, and includes foods in moderate proportions. Personalized meal plans including the caloric requirements for your own needs can be provided by a registered dietitian. Should you need assistance with finding a registered dietitian in your area, you can contact the American Dietetic Association hotline at ✆ 800-366-1655.

## Day 1

- **Breakfast:** ½ cup apple juice, 2 slices French toast, 1 tablespoon light maple syrup, 1 cup low-fat milk
- **Lunch:** Sub sandwich (1 ounce deli-sliced turkey, 1 ounce deli-sliced roast beef, 1 ounce deli-sliced cheese, 1 small bun, 2 lettuce/tomato slices, and 1 tablespoon light mayonnaise), 4 baby carrot sticks, 1 medium apple
- **Dinner:** 3 ounces veal chop, ½ cup mashed potatoes, 2 spears steamed broccoli, ½ cup applesauce
- **Snack:** ¾ cup low-fat vanilla yogurt, ¼ cup low-fat granola

## Day 2

- **Breakfast:** ½ cup orange juice, ¾ cup bran flakes with raisins, 1 cup low-fat milk
- **Lunch:** Chicken salad on pita (consisting of 3 ounces chopped chicken, 1 tablespoon light mayonnaise, ¼ cup cut-up grapes, ¼ cup water chestnuts, 1 whole-wheat pita bread), one wedge of watermelon (2 inches by 4 inches)
- **Snack:** 2 squares of graham crackers, 1 cup low-fat milk
- **Dinner:** 3 ounces poached fish fillets, Parmesan noodles (½ cup wide noodles, 1 teaspoon Parmesan cheese, 1 teaspoon light margarine), ½ cup steamed zucchini, 1 cup tossed salad with 1 tablespoon low-fat salad dressing, 1 dinner roll

## Day 3

- **Breakfast:** ½ grapefruit, ½ whole-wheat English muffin with 1 teaspoon fruit spread, 1 cup low-fat milk
- **Lunch:** Hamburger (3 ounces hamburger patty, 2 lettuce/tomato slices, 3 pickle slices, 1 bun), 1 ounce pretzel sticks, 1 peach
- **Snack:** ½ cup Bing cherries
- **Dinner:** Chicken stir-fry (consisting of 3 ounces chicken strips, ¼ cup broccoli, ¼ cup red pepper slices, ⅛ cup mushrooms, ⅛ cup bamboo shoots, 2 teaspoons soy sauce), ½ cup steamed white rice, 1 fortune cookie
- **Snack:** Creamsicle shake (½ cup orange sherbet, ½ cup low-fat vanilla frozen yogurt)

## Day 4

- **Breakfast:** ½ cup pineapple/grapefruit juice, 1 sesame bagel with 1 teaspoon light margarine and 1 teaspoon fruit spread
- **Lunch:** ½ cup low-fat cottage cheese, tuna/pasta salad (3 ounces tuna, 2 tablespoons light mayonnaise, ½ cup pasta, 2 to 3 lettuce leaves, 5 or 6 cherry tomatoes, ½ cup red pepper slices), ¼ cantaloupe
- **Snack:** 10 to 12 grapes
- **Dinner:** 3 ounces London broil, ½ cup brown rice, 4 asparagus spears, 1 breadstick, 1 teaspoon margarine
- **Snack:** 4 vanilla wafers, 1 cup low-fat milk

## Day 5

- **Breakfast:** ½ cup cranberry juice, 2 scrambled eggs, 2 pieces whole-wheat toast with 1 teaspoon fruit spread, 1 cup low-fat milk
- **Lunch:** 1 cup tomato soup, 1 cup spinach salad with ½ cup strawberry slices and 1 tablespoon poppy seed dressing, 1 hard roll
- **Snack:** 1 cup carrot/cucumber slices, 2 tablespoons low-fat dip (peppercorn ranch)
- **Dinner:** 4 ounces grilled salmon, 1 baked potato with 1 teaspoon low-fat sour cream, ½ cup green beans almandine, 1 (2-inch) square of cornbread
- **Snack:** ½ cup low-fat frozen yogurt, 1 small tangerine

## Day 6

- **Breakfast:** 1 orange, ¾ cup bran flakes, 1 cup low-fat milk
- **Lunch:** 1 cup vegetarian bean chili, 5 crackers, 1 cup leafy green salad with 1 tablespoon low-fat dressing, 1 French roll with 1 teaspoon low-fat margarine
- **Dinner:** 1-inch slice ground turkey meat loaf, 1 medium ear of corn on the cob, ½ cup steamed pea pods, ½ cup fruit cocktail
- **Snack:** 1-inch slice angel food cake, ½ cup fresh raspberries, 1 cup low-fat milk

## Day 7

- **Breakfast:** ½ cup tomato juice, 1 low-fat multigrain bar, 1 cup low-fat milk
- **Lunch:** Chicken/rice salad in tomato (2 ounces chopped chicken, 1 tablespoon light mayonnaise, ¼ cup cooked rice, ½ cup shredded zucchini/broccoli/carrots, 1 tomato), 2 small clementines
- **Snack:** 5 mini or 1 large rice cake, 1 cup low-fat milk
- **Dinner:** 3 ounces sliced turkey, ½ cup stuffing with chopped celery, 1 tablespoon cranberry sauce, ½ cup French-cut green beans, 1 slice sourdough bread, 1 teaspoon light margarine
- **Snack:** 1 apple, 2 gingersnaps

## Day 8

- **Breakfast:** ½ cup pineapple juice, 1 poached egg, 1 biscuit, 1 teaspoon light margarine, 1 teaspoon fruit spread, 1 cup low-fat milk
- **Snack:** 1 banana
- **Lunch:** Roast beef sandwich (2 ounces roast beef, 2 slices rye bread, 1 teaspoon mustard), marinated cucumbers (½ cup sliced cucumbers, 1 tablespoon low-fat Italian dressing), 1 ounce baked chips
- **Dinner:** Chicken tacos (3 ounces chopped chicken, ½ cup shredded lettuce, 2 tablespoons shredded low-fat Cheddar cheese, ¼ cup chopped tomatoes, 1 tablespoon salsa, 2 taco shells)
- **Snack:** ½ cup sliced strawberries with 1 teaspoon confectioners' sugar

## Day 9

- **Breakfast:** ½ grapefruit, ½ cup cooked oatmeal, 1 cup low-fat milk
- **Snack:** ½ bagel, 1 teaspoon fruit spread
- **Lunch:** Stuffed baked potato (1 medium baked potato, ½ cup steamed broccoli, 1 tablespoon shredded cheese, 1 teaspoon light margarine), ½ cup fresh fruit salad
- **Dinner:** 3 ounces pork chops, ½ cup wild rice, ½ cup steamed peas and carrots, 1 cup tossed spinach salad with 1 tablespoon low-fat dressing, 1 dinner roll, 1 teaspoon low-fat margarine
- **Snack:** Fruit smoothie (1 cup low-fat vanilla yogurt, ½ cup frozen banana and/or berries)

## Day 10

- **Breakfast:** ½ cup orange juice, 1 blueberry muffin, 1 cup low-fat milk
- **Lunch:** Asian chicken salad (1 cup chopped lettuce, ½ cup chopped chicken, 6 cherry tomatoes, ½ cucumber sliced, ½ cup crunchy noodles, 2 tablespoons Asian salad dressing), 1 sourdough roll
- **Snack:** 1 medium nectarine
- **Dinner:** Baked fish (3 ounces fish fillet, 1 tablespoon bread crumb coating, 1 teaspoon light margarine, 1 teaspoon lemon juice), parsley potatoes (½ cup chopped red potatoes, 1 teaspoon light margarine, ½ teaspoon parsley), vegetable stir-fry medley (½ cup sliced green and red peppers, ¼ cup onions, ¼ cup broccoli)
- **Snack:** 1 cup low-fat yogurt

## Day 11

- **Breakfast:** ½ cup white grape juice, 2 slices raisin bread, 1 teaspoon light margarine
- **Lunch:** Cottage cheese/fruit platter (¾ cup low-fat cottage cheese, ½ cup cantaloupe cubes, ½ cup honeydew melon cubes, ½ cup watermelon cubes, ½ cup pineapple cubes, ¼ cup mango cubes), 1 hard roll with 1 teaspoon light margarine
- **Dinner:** Spaghetti with meat sauce (3 ounces cooked lean ground beef, ½ cup spaghetti sauce, ½ cup spaghetti noodles), Caesar salad (1 cup romaine lettuce, ¼ cup croutons, 1 tablespoon low-fat Caesar dressing), garlic bread (1 slice French bread, 1 teaspoon margarine, 1 teaspoon chopped garlic or garlic powder), ½ cup sliced peaches

## Day 12

- **Breakfast:** ½ cup grape juice, 1 cup multigrain oat cereal, 1 cup low-fat milk
- **Lunch:** Tuna melt (3 ounces tuna, 1 tablespoon light mayonnaise, 1 ounce mozzarella cheese, 1 English muffin), 4 to 5 baby carrots, ½ cup pineapple slices
- **Snack:** 1 ounce pretzel sticks, 1 cup low-fat chocolate milk
- **Dinner:** 3 ounces roasted Cornish hen, 1 medium baked sweet potato, ½ cup steamed baby peas, ½ cup rainbow sherbet
- **Snack:** 2 cups air-popped popcorn, ½ cup orange juice

## Day 13

- **Breakfast:** ½ cup fruit cocktail, 1 hardboiled egg, 1 slice whole-wheat toast with 1 teaspoon light margarine and 1 teaspoon fruit spread, 1 cup low-fat milk
- **Snack:** 1 tangerine
- **Lunch:** Pizza bread (½ French roll, 2 tablespoons pizza sauce, 2 ounces mozzarella cheese), 6 cherry tomatoes, ½ cucumber, sliced
- **Snack:** 5 vanilla wafers, 1 cup low-fat milk
- **Dinner:** Chicken kabobs (3 ounces grilled chicken, ½ onion cut into wedges, ½ green pepper cut into wedges, ½ red pepper cut into wedges, 6 whole mushrooms), ½ cup steamed brown rice, 1 cup Bibb lettuce salad with 1 tablespoon low-fat dressing
- **Snack:** 1 medium pear

## Day 14

- **Breakfast:** ½ cup grapefruit wedges, 1 bran muffin with 1 teaspoon margarine, 1 cup low-fat milk
- **Lunch:** Vegetarian omelet (2 eggs, ¼ cup chopped tomatoes, ¼ cup mushrooms, ¼ cup zucchini), 1 whole-wheat bagel with 2 teaspoons light margarine, 1 cup low-fat milk
- **Snack:** 1 medium apple
- **Dinner:** 3 ounces grilled salmon, ½ cup potato wedges, spinach/ orange salad (1 cup spinach, ¼ cup mandarin orange sections, 1 tablespoon low-fat dressing), 1 dinner roll with 1 teaspoon light margarine
- **Snack:** 5 mini or 1 large rice cake

As you can see from the preceding examples, it does help to plan meals and snacks ahead of time. If you plan ahead you will be better prepared to shop and cook to meet your needs. Not only does it help to plan main courses, it's a good idea for side dishes and snacks as well. Developing a weekly or biweekly cycle menu plan can assist you in making the right choices for you and your family. Why not start today?

## CHAPTER 19

# *Keeping Your Personal Records and Diet Diary*

**B**efore beginning any weight-loss program, it is recommended that you visit your doctor for a complete physical. Be sure to tell her about your plans to reduce your food intake and improve on your exercise routine. It is also a good idea to make note of your personal height, weight, blood pressure, and total cholesterol levels.

# Your Records

The following records offer you a starting point at which you began your program. Note the date and other relevant information. Periodically (once per month) update your list with any new data.

Date

Height

Weight

Blood Pressure

Total Cholesterol Levels

     HDL

     LDL

Body Mass Index

My Body Measurements

     Chest/Bust

     Waist

     Hips

     Upper Thigh

     Calf

     Upper Arm

     Lower Arm

     Waist-to-Hip Ratio

     Apple versus Pear Shaped

# Setting Goals

Again, I encourage you to set your long- and short-term goals before you begin your program. Here you can determine what you hope to accomplish. By writing down this information, you make a commitment to yourself to continue.

List major problem areas regarding eating, exercise, and food-related behaviors:

1. _____
2. _____
3. _____
4. _____
5. _____

List long-term goals (those you would like to accomplish in six months to one year from now):

1. _____
2. _____
3. _____
4. _____
5. _____

List short-term goals (goals that you wish to accomplish one week at a time):

1. _____
2. _____
3. _____
4. _____
5. _____

# MILESTONES

| Date | Accomplishment | Reward | How You Felt |
|------|----------------|--------|--------------|
|      |                |        |              |

# Creating Your Diet/Exercise Diary

The food and exercise diary is the most effective tool for those seeking to lose and maintain weight. Studies have proved those individuals who keep accurate records not only lose more weight but keep it off too. Why?

By recording food intake, exercise patterns, and behaviors associated with eating, you get the following benefits:

- You realize just what you eat, how much, and how often. You may also even be able to determine triggers that cause you to overeat.
- You can identify problem areas, such as excessive portions, frequent snacking, or lack of activity, that you wish to tackle.
- You become more disciplined with your lifestyle patterns. You will think twice about overeating, skipping meals, or missing your workout.
- You can identify moods and situations that cause excess eating. By noting your hunger level, moods, and amounts you eat, you can determine whether various moods result in overeating.
- You are motivated to strive toward your goals.
- You learn to plan ahead.

## How to Best Use Your Diet/Exercise Diary

Set your daily goals. Fill in the following Food Guide Pyramid. Refer to Chapter 6 for additional assistance.

Complete a new diary form for each day. Record day, date, time, mood, hunger level, food eaten, and how much as indicated. Be accurate. Weigh and measure food if necessary. Be sure to include all snacks and beverages, too.

As you list your food intake, mark off the appropriate food group box in the personal check-off Food Guide Pyramid that follows. Here, you can compare your actual intake to your daily goals.

Record daily exercise/activity over and above daily routines. Aim for an extra thirty to fifty minutes each day.

At the end of the day, record some comments to help you continue tomorrow. Your comments can relate to feelings, accomplishments, difficulties, and so on.

# DIET/EXERCISE DIARY

## Daily goals

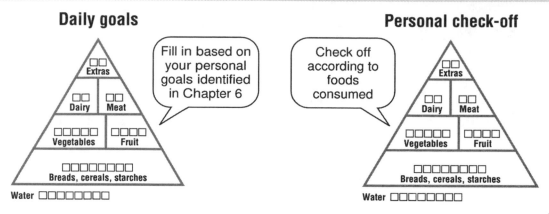

Fill in based on your personal goals identified in Chapter 6

## Personal check-off

Check off according to foods consumed

Extras

Dairy    Meat

Vegetables    Fruit

Breads, cereals, starches

Water ☐☐☐☐☐☐☐☐

Day _____    Date _____

| Time* | Mood** | Hunger level*** | Food eaten## | How much### |
|-------|--------|-----------------|--------------|-------------|
|       |        |                 |              |             |

\* Time = time of day at which you have eaten
** Mood = how you feel (happy, sad, frustrated, stressed, nervous, etc.)
*** Hunger level = how hungry you are. Rate 1–5 (1 not hungry to 5 famished)
## Food eaten = all food consumed. Be specific.
### How much = portion size. Be specific.

### Daily exercise

| Time | Type of activity | Duration |
|------|------------------|----------|
|      |                  |          |

### Daily comments

| (indicate here how you feel, how you did, how well you would like to improve) |
|---|
|  |

# DIET/EXERCISE DIARY

## Daily goals

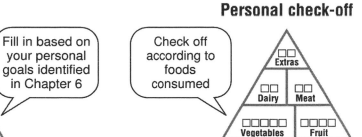

```
      ☐☐
      Extras
   ☐☐      ☐☐
   Dairy    Meat
  ☐☐☐☐☐   ☐☐☐☐
  Vegetables   Fruit
    ☐☐☐☐☐☐☐☐
 Breads, cereals, starches
```
Water ☐☐☐☐☐☐☐☐

## Personal check-off

Check off according to foods consumed

```
      ☐☐
      Extras
   ☐☐      ☐☐
   Dairy    Meat
  ☐☐☐☐☐   ☐☐☐☐
  Vegetables   Fruit
    ☐☐☐☐☐☐☐☐
 Breads, cereals, starches
```
Water ☐☐☐☐☐☐☐☐

Day _____     Date _____

| Time* | Mood** | Hunger level*** | Food eaten## | How much### |
|-------|--------|-----------------|--------------|-------------|
|       |        |                 |              |             |
|       |        |                 |              |             |
|       |        |                 |              |             |
|       |        |                 |              |             |

\* Time = time of day at which you have eaten
\*\* Mood = how you feel (happy, sad, frustrated, stressed, nervous, etc.)
\*\*\* Hunger level = how hungry you are. Rate 1–5 (1 not hungry to 5 famished)
## Food eaten = all food consumed. Be specific.
### How much = portion size. Be specific.

### Daily exercise

| Time | Type of activity | Duration |
|------|------------------|----------|
|      |                  |          |

### Daily comments

| (indicate here how you feel, how you did, how well you would like to improve) |
|---|
|  |

# DIET/EXERCISE DIARY

## Daily goals

☐☐
**Extras**

☐☐ ☐☐
**Dairy** **Meat**

☐☐☐☐☐ ☐☐☐☐
**Vegetables** **Fruit**

☐☐☐☐☐☐☐☐
**Breads, cereals, starches**

Water ☐☐☐☐☐☐☐☐

> Fill in based on your personal goals identified in Chapter 6

## Personal check-off

> Check off according to foods consumed

☐☐
**Extras**

☐☐ ☐☐
**Dairy** **Meat**

☐☐☐☐☐ ☐☐☐☐
**Vegetables** **Fruit**

☐☐☐☐☐☐☐☐
**Breads, cereals, starches**

Water ☐☐☐☐☐☐☐☐

Day _____     Date _____

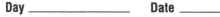

| Time* | Mood** | Hunger level*** | Food eaten## | How much### |
|-------|--------|-----------------|--------------|-------------|
|       |        |                 |              |             |
|       |        |                 |              |             |
|       |        |                 |              |             |
|       |        |                 |              |             |
|       |        |                 |              |             |

\* Time = time of day at which you have eaten
** Mood = how you feel (happy, sad, frustrated, stressed, nervous, etc.)
*** Hunger level = how hungry you are. Rate 1–5 (1 not hungry to 5 famished)
## Food eaten = all food consumed. Be specific.
### How much = portion size. Be specific.

### Daily exercise

| Time | Type of activity | Duration |
|------|------------------|----------|
|      |                  |          |

### Daily comments

| (indicate here how you feel, how you did, how well you would like to improve) |
|---|
|  |

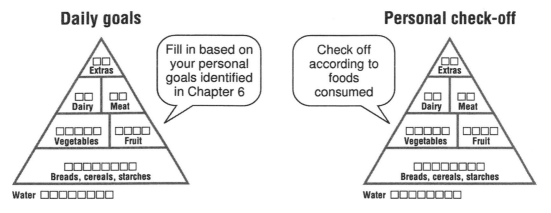

**Daily goals**

Fill in based on your personal goals identified in Chapter 6

**Personal check-off**

Check off according to foods consumed

Day _____ Date _____

| Time* | Mood** | Hunger level*** | Food eaten## | How much### |
|-------|--------|-----------------|--------------|-------------|
|       |        |                 |              |             |
|       |        |                 |              |             |
|       |        |                 |              |             |
|       |        |                 |              |             |
|       |        |                 |              |             |
|       |        |                 |              |             |

\* Time = time of day at which you have eaten
** Mood = how you feel (happy, sad, frustrated, stressed, nervous, etc.)
*** Hunger level = how hungry you are. Rate 1–5 (1 not hungry to 5 famished)
## Food eaten = all food consumed. Be specific.
### How much = portion size. Be specific.

### Daily exercise

| Time | Type of activity | Duration |
|------|------------------|----------|
|      |                  |          |

### Daily comments

| **(indicate here how you feel, how you did, how well you would like to improve)** |
|---|
|  |

## DIET/EXERCISE DIARY

### Daily goals

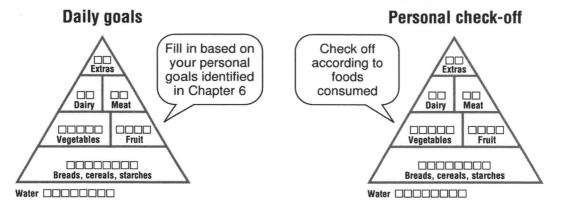

Fill in based on your personal goals identified in Chapter 6

### Personal check-off

Check off according to foods consumed

Day _____  Date _____

| Time* | Mood** | Hunger level*** | Food eaten## | How much### |
|-------|--------|-----------------|--------------|-------------|
|       |        |                 |              |             |
|       |        |                 |              |             |
|       |        |                 |              |             |
|       |        |                 |              |             |

\* Time = time of day at which you have eaten
\** Mood = how you feel (happy, sad, frustrated, stressed, nervous, etc.)
\*** Hunger level = how hungry you are. Rate 1–5 (1 not hungry to 5 famished)
## Food eaten = all food consumed. Be specific.
### How much = portion size. Be specific.

### Daily exercise

| Time | Type of activity | Duration |
|------|------------------|----------|
|      |                  |          |

### Daily comments

| (indicate here how you feel, how you did, how well you would like to improve) |
|---|
|   |

## EVALUATING RESULTS

At the end of each week, note your results on the Weight-Loss Chart. Here you should plot the number of pounds lost based on the particular week. As the weeks move on, you will be able to visually see how well you are doing.

## WEIGHT LOSS CHART

| POUNDS LOST | 1 | 2 | 3 | 4 | 5 | 6 | 7 | 8 | 9 | 10 |
|---|---|---|---|---|---|---|---|---|---|---|
| 25 | | | | | | | | | | |
| 24 | | | | | | | | | | |
| 23 | | | | | | | | | | |
| 22 | | | | | | | | | | |
| 21 | | | | | | | | | | |
| 20 | | | | | | | | | | |
| 19 | | | | | | | | | | |
| 18 | | | | | | | | | | |
| 17 | | | | | | | | | | |
| 16 | | | | | | | | | | |
| 15 | | | | | | | | | | |
| 14 | | | | | | | | | | |
| 13 | | | | | | | | | | |
| 12 | | | | | | | | | | |
| 11 | | | | | | | | | | |
| 10 | | | | | | | | | | |
| 9 | | | | | | | | | | |
| 8 | | | | | | | | | | |
| 7 | | | | | | | | | | |
| 6 | | | | | | | | | | |
| 5 | | | | | | | | | | |
| 4 | | | | | | | | | | |
| 3 | | | | | | | | | | |
| 2 | | | | | | | | | | |
| 1 | | | | | | | | | | |
| | 1 | 2 | 3 | 4 | 5 | 6 | 7 | 8 | 9 | 10 |

WEEK

Each week, make a dot indicating the number of pounds you've lost. Connect the dots to illustrate your progress.

Goal-setting, along with use of the diet/exercise diary, is the most effective means of motivating yourself and monitoring your status and progress. Nutrition professionals agree that this type of process works well with people of all ages and with all parties involved. It allows users to accurately keep records and allows those monitoring the progress to evaluate problems effectively.

Give your diary a try. Keep with it. Observe your success and determine for yourself how and why this method works.

Good luck and healthy eating!

CHAPTER 20

# Recipes for Dieting Success

The following recipes are a sampling of those you may wish to add to your personal collection. These are shared with you to give you ideas on expanding your meals and snacks to include a wide variety of choices.

# Vegetable Omelet

**Serves 2**
½ vegetable, 1 meat

Calories per serving: 140

Protein: 10 grams

Carbohydrates: 5 grams

Fat: 9 grams

Fiber: 1 gram

**To save 50 calories and 5 grams of fat per serving, substitute 2 egg whites and 1 whole egg for the 3 eggs.**

ᔆ

*3 large eggs*
*2 tablespoons low-fat milk*
*salt and pepper to taste*
*1 teaspoon light margarine*
*1 scallion, finely chopped*
*¼ cup finely chopped red*
*   pepper*

*¼ cup finely chopped green*
*   pepper*
*1 teaspoon fresh parsley*

1. In a medium bowl, beat together the eggs, milk, salt, and pepper.
2. Melt margarine in skillet over high heat. Add scallion and peppers. Sauté for 2 to 3 minutes or until the vegetables begin to soften. Pour the egg mixture into the skillet over the vegetables. Cook for about 30 seconds, until the eggs begin to set. Use a metal spatula to lift the eggs, and tilt the pan to allow the uncooked eggs to flow to the edges. When the top portion of the eggs begins to set, fold the egg mixture in half to form the omelet. Transfer omelet to serving plate. Sprinkle with fresh parsley.

*Recipes have been analyzed using the Food Processor II Nutrition Software. Nutrition information has been listed for total calories and grams of protein, carbohydrates, fat, and fiber per serving. (Optional ingredients and additional suggestions and substitutions are not included in the analysis.) Figures are rounded to the nearest value. Also provided are the dietary exchanges to help you determine to which food group each recipe contributes. All of this information is provided to help you determine the best options for your personal needs.*

# Blueberry Crumb Muffins

¼ cup margarine, softened
⅔ cup sugar
2 eggs
½ cup low-fat milk
1 teaspoon vanilla
2 cups flour
2 teaspoons baking powder
dash salt
1½ cups fresh blueberries,
   rinsed

## Crumb Topping:

¼ cup sugar
¼ cup flour
1 teaspoon cinnamon
2 tablespoons margarine,
   softened

---

**Yields 1 dozen**
**1 bread, ½ fruit, 2 fats**

Calories per serving: 216

Protein: 4 grams

Carbohydrates: 35 grams

Fat: 7 grams

Fiber: 1 gram

---

To save 43 calories and 2 grams of fat per serving, try the muffins without the topping.

∾

---

1. Preheat oven to 350 degrees. Spray a muffin tin pan with cooking spray.
2. Using an electric mixer, cream together the ¼ cup margarine and ⅔ cup sugar. Add eggs, milk, and vanilla. Carefully add the flour, baking powder, and salt to batter, combining until just mixed and moistened. Fold in the blueberries using a wooden spoon or rubber spatula. Pour batter into prepared pan to a third of the way from the top.
3. Prepare crumb topping. In a small bowl combine the sugar, flour, and cinnamon. Add margarine and mix together using a pastry cutter or fork, until the mixture is crumbly. Sprinkle crumb topping over the tops of the batter.
4. Bake muffins for 20 to 25 minutes or until light brown and a toothpick inserted into the center of the muffins comes out clean. Cool before serving.

# Yogurt-Peach Smoothie

**Serves 2**
1 fruit, 1 dairy, 1 fat

Calories per serving: 186

Protein: 8 grams

Carbohydrates: 34 grams

Fat: 3 grams

Fiber: 1 gram

Try this smoothie with different types of frozen fruits, too—like blueberries, strawberries, and bananas.

*1 (8-ounce) container low-fat vanilla yogurt*

*½ cup low-fat milk*
*½ cup frozen peach slices*

Combine all ingredients in blender. Cover. Blend until smooth.

# Orange-Banana Freeze

**Serves 4**
1½ fruit

Calories: 139

Protein: 4 grams

Carbohydrates: 30 grams

Fat: 1 gram

Fiber: 1 gram

This delicious frozen beverage will remind you of a Dreamsicle pop.

*1 (6-ounce) can undiluted frozen orange juice concentrate*
*¾ cup water*
*1 (8-ounce) container low-fat vanilla yogurt*

*1 small banana, peeled and frozen*

Combine all ingredients in blender. Cover. Blend until smooth.

# Cranberry Bran Muffins

1 cup flour
1½ teaspoon baking powder
½ teaspoon baking soda
½ teaspoon cinnamon
¼ teaspoon nutmeg
2 cups (100 percent) all-bran cereal

1½ cups low-fat milk
⅓ cup brown sugar
1 egg, lightly beaten
½ cup applesauce
½ cup dried cranberries

**Yields 1 dozen**
1 bread, ½ fruit

Calories: 130

Protein: 4 grams

Carbohydrates: 28 grams

Fat: 1.5 grams

Fiber: 4 grams

Try mini-muffin tins and make 3 dozen at 43 calories and .5 grams of fat per mini-muffin.

1. Preheat oven to 375 degrees. Spray muffin tin with cooking spray.
2. In large bowl, combine flour, baking powder, baking soda, cinnamon, and nutmeg.
3. In another medium bowl, combine bran cereal, milk, and brown sugar. Set aside for several minutes. Add beaten egg, applesauce, and cranberries. Mix well.
4. Pour cereal mixture into flour mixture. Stir until just moistened; batter will be slightly lumpy. Do not over mix.
5. Pour batter into prepared muffin tin pan to a third of the way from the top. Bake 20 minutes or until browned. A toothpick inserted into the center of the muffins should come out clean. Cool before serving.

# Very Berry Smoothie

1 (8-ounce) container low-fat vanilla yogurt
½ cup low-fat milk

¼ cup frozen strawberries
¼ cup frozen blueberries

Combine all ingredients in blender. Cover. Blend until smooth.

# Fruit Wrap

2 (8-inch) flour tortillas
2 teaspoons low-fat cream cheese
2 teaspoons honey
2 tablespoons raisins

1 small apple, peeled and finely chopped
1 teaspoon sugar
½ teaspoon cinnamon

1. Spread cream cheese and honey over tortillas. Top with raisins and chopped apples. Sprinkle sugar and cinnamon over the fruit.
2. Roll tortillas. Secure with toothpick, if desired.

# Grilled Vegetable Sandwich

1½ pounds of assorted fresh
   vegetables (red, green,
   yellow bell peppers; mushrooms; zucchini; onion; eggplant), thinly sliced
1 tablespoons red wine vinegar
   or balsamic vinegar

2 tablespoons olive or
   vegetable oil
¼ teaspoon dried basil leaves
2 pita breads, cut in half

1. In a large bowl, combine vegetable with vinegar, oil, and basil. Toss.
   Place vegetables on a grill rack or wrapped in aluminum foil and
   place over hot coals on a grill or in a 350 degree oven. Cook about
   20 to 30 minutes until vegetables are tender.
2. Stuff each pita half with vegetable mixture. Serve warm.

| **Serves 4** |
| --- |
| **1 bread, 2 vegetables** |
| Calories per serving: 132 |
| Protein: 5 grams |
| Carbohydrates: 27 grams |
| Fat: 1 gram |
| Fiber: 3 grams |

Be creative. Try other vegetables of your liking and even different types of breads like focaccia and French loaves.

 ～

# Turkey Veggie Wrap

2 tablespoons light salad
   dressing of choice
4 (8-inch) flour tortillas
½ pound deli-sliced turkey
1 cup shredded lettuce

½ cup cooked corn or 1 ear
   corn-on-the-cob, cooked, then
   corn removed
¼ cup chopped red bell
   pepper

1. Spread salad dressing over tortillas. Layer each tortilla with turkey
   slices, shredded lettuce, corn, and red pepper. Roll tortilla and secure
   with toothpicks until ready to eat.

| **Serves 4** |
| --- |
| **1 bread, 1 vegetable, 1 meat** |
| Calories per serving: 203 |
| Protein: 15 grams |
| Carbohydrates: 24 grams |
| Fat: 6 grams |
| Fiber: 3 grams |

For a change, add 1 tablespoon of shredded cheese. If you are concerned about the fat, reduce or remove the dressing.

 ～

# Thai Lettuce Wraps

**Serves 4**
1 bread, ½ vegetable,
½ meat, ½ fat

Calories per serving: 191

Protein: 10 grams

Carbohydrates: 32 grams

Fat: 2 grams

Fiber: 1 gram

For extra crunch, add ¼ cup chopped peanuts to the sauce. This will add an additional 51 calories and 4 grams of fat per serving.

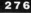

1 boneless, skinless chicken breast, chopped into small pieces
1 teaspoon vegetable oil
2 tablespoons soy sauce
2 tablespoons chopped onion
1 tablespoon sugar
1 tablespoon minced cilantro
1½ teaspoons lime juice
1 clove garlic, minced
½ teaspoon grated ginger
¼ teaspoon red pepper flakes
2 cups cooked rice
8 large lettuce leaves

1. In large skillet, heat oil. Add chicken strips. Sauté chicken until done and no longer pink.
2. In large bowl, combine soy sauce, onion, sugar, cilantro, lime juice, garlic, ginger, and red pepper. Mix well. Add cooked chicken. Place into the refrigerator for ½ hour.
3. Prepare rice according to package directions.
4. Place lettuce leaves onto a serving plate. Place rice in a large bowl and chicken mixture in another bowl. Using lettuce leaves as wraps, top each one with about 2 tablespoons of the warm rice and a small spoonful of the chicken mixture (along with sauce). Wrap up and serve immediately.

# Spinach Crustless Quiche

2 eggs
2 egg whites
½ cup low-fat milk
1 (10-ounce) package frozen
　chopped spinach, thawed
　and drained
½ cup chopped green onions
salt and pepper to taste
½ cup part-skim, shredded
　mozzarella cheese

1. Preheat oven to 375 degrees. Spray 8-inch round quiche pan with cooking spray.
2. In large bowl, mix together the eggs, egg whites, and milk. Add the spinach, onions, salt and pepper. Pour into prepared pan. Sprinkle with shredded cheese.
3. Bake 30 to 35 minutes or until quiche is light brown and cooked throughout. Cool slightly before serving.

**Serves 6**
½ vegetable, ½ meat,
½ fat

Calories per serving: 81

Protein: 8 grams

Carbohydrates: 4 grams

Fat: 4 grams

Fiber: 1 gram

If you prefer, try a prepared crust, but beware of the extra 133 calories and 8 grams of fat you will add per serving.

# Grilled Cheese and Tomato Sandwich

2 teaspoons margarine
4 slices fresh sourdough bread
1 tomato, thinly sliced
2 slices Swiss or Muenster
　cheese

1. Spread margarine over one side of each bread slice. On unbuttered side, layer tomatoes and cheese. Top with other slice of bread, the buttered side out.
2. Heat large skillet. Place sandwiches in skillet. Cook for about 2 minutes on each side, until golden brown.

**Serves 2**
2 breads, ½ vegetable,
1 dairy, 1 fat

Calories per serving: 288

Protein: 13 grams

Carbohydrates: 27 grams

Fat: 14 grams

Fiber: 2 grams

Opt for low-fat cheese and reduce your calories by 57 and fat by 8 grams per serving.

# Tomato Pesto Pizza

**Serves 8**
1 bread, ½ dairy, ½ fat

Calories per serving: 154

Protein: 7 grams

Carbohydrates: 18 grams

Fat: 5 grams

Fiber: 1 gram

To jazz up your pizza
and up the fiber, too,
add fresh peppers
(green and red),
onions, mushrooms,
broccoli, and any other
favorite vegetables.

*1 prepared pizza crust*
*2 tablespoons prepared pesto*
*sauce*
*2 large tomatoes, finely chopped*

*2 garlic cloves, minced*
*1 cup part-skim, shredded*
*mozzarella cheese*

1. Preheat oven to 450 degrees.
2. Place pizza crust on baking sheet. Spread pesto sauce over the pizza crust. Top with chopped tomatoes, garlic, and mozzarella cheese. Bake 10 to 12 minutes or until cheese is melted and lightly browned on top.

# Cheesy Tortilla Soup

**Serves 4**
1 vegetable, ½ fat

Calories: 75

Protein: 5 grams

Carbohydrates: 12 grams

Fat: 2 grams

Fiber: 2.5 grams

Try a cup with a half
of sandwich for a
quick (and light) lunch
or dinner.

*1 onion, diced*
*2 garlic cloves, minced*
*2 (14-ounce) cans vegetable or*
*chicken broth*
*1 (14.5-ounce) can diced*
*tomatoes*

*1 tablespoon chopped cilantro*
*1 teaspoon cumin*
*1 teaspoon chili powder*
*¼ cup low-fat shredded*
*Cheddar cheese*
*4–5 tortilla chips*

1. In large saucepan, sauté onion and garlic in 1 to 2 tablespoons of the broth until tender. Add remaining broth, tomatoes, cilantro (if desired), cumin, and chili powder. Simmer for 20 minutes.
2. Strain and reserve liquid from soup. Purée remaining vegetables in blender. Return to strained soup. Mix well.
3. Pour soup into serving bowls. Top with cheese and tortilla chips to serve.

# Pocket Sandwich

1 pita bread
1 (6-ounce) can tuna, packed
   in water
1 tablespoon light mayonnaise

$1/4$ cup grapes, sliced
$1/4$ cup shredded Cheddar
   cheese
$1/4$ cup chopped celery

1. Cut pita bread in half to make 2 separate pockets.
2. In a small bowl, combine remaining ingredients. Mix well. Stuff into pita pockets. Serve immediately.

---

**Serves 2**
**1 bread, ½ fruit,**
**1 meat, 1 fat**

| | |
|---|---|
| Calories: 272 | |
| Protein: 28 grams | |
| Carbohydrates: 22 grams | |
| Fat: 7 grams | |
| Fiber: 1 gram | |

Try low-fat Cheddar cheese and reduce calories by 32 and fat by almost 4 grams per serving.

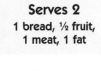

---

# Cool Cucumber Salad

1 cucumber, peeled and thinly
   sliced
$1/2$ teaspoon dill
$1/4$ teaspoon salt

$1/4$ cup rice vinegar
1 tablespoon sugar
Dash pepper

1. Place cucumber slices in a medium bowl.
2. In a small bowl or jar, combine remaining ingredients. Mix well. Pour dressing over cucumbers. Toss well.

---

**Serves 6**
**½ vegetable**

| | |
|---|---|
| Calories: 13 | |
| Protein: 0 | |
| Carbohydrates: 3 grams | |
| Fat: 0 | |
| Fiber: 0 | |

This refreshing side dish makes a wonderful accompaniment to many chicken, fish, and beef dishes.

# Soothing Tomato Soup

**Serves 6**
**2 vegetables**

Calories per serving: 79

Protein: 2 grams

Carbohydrates: 13 grams

Fat: 3 grams

Fiber: 3 grams

Try this soup with fresh bread or crackers as a light meal. It's sure to fill you up.

1  tablespoon vegetable oil
1  garlic clove, minced
1  cup finely chopped onion
3  pounds ripe tomatoes,
    peeled, cored, and chopped
1  teaspoon salt
½  teaspoon pepper
½  teaspoon chopped basil

1. In a large saucepan or Dutch oven, heat oil. Add garlic and onion. Sauté 3 to 4 minutes, until onion is tender. Add tomatoes, salt, and pepper. Heat to boiling. Reduce heat, cover, and simmer for 20 minutes. Remove from heat. Cool slightly.
2. Take 1 cup of the tomato mixture at a time and pour into a blender. Blend until smooth. Pour out into large saucepan, and continue until all of the tomato mixture is well blended. Heat to warm before serving. Sprinkle with chopped basil.

# Vegetable Barley Soup

**Serves 6**
**2 vegetables, 1 meat**

Calories per serving: 139

Protein: 5 grams

Carbohydrates: 31 grams

Fat: 1 gram

Fiber: 7 grams

To make a full meal, add some leftover cooked chicken.

2  (14-ounce) cans vegetable or
    chicken broth
1  teaspoon salt
½  teaspoon pepper
¼  teaspoon oregano
1  cup chopped carrot
1  cup chopped celery
1  cup chopped potato
½  cup chopped onion
½  cup chopped green pepper
½  cup uncooked pearl barley
1  (28-ounce) can diced toma-
    toes, not drained

In a large saucepan or Dutch oven, combine broth, salt, pepper, and oregano. Heat to boiling. Add remaining ingredients. Reduce heat. Simmer for 20 to 30 minutes or until vegetables are tender.

# Zesty Broccoli Cheese Soup

2 (14-ounce) cans vegetable or
   chicken broth
1½ cups water
1 (10-ounce) can diced tomatoes (can also use diced
   tomatoes with spicy peppers)

2 (10-ounce) packages frozen
   chopped broccoli
1 cup low-fat Cheddar cheese,
   cubed or shredded

1. In a large saucepan or Dutch oven, combine broth, water, tomatoes, and broccoli. Heat to boiling. Reduce heat and simmer 20 to 30 minutes or until broccoli is tender-soft. Remove from heat.
2. Take 1 cup of the soup mixture at a time and purée in blender or food processor until smooth. Return puréed soup to saucepan.
3. Add cheese cubes to saucepan. Stir until melted and soup is thickened.

| **Serves 8** |
| 1 vegetable, ½ dairy |
| --- |
| Calories per serving: 89 |
| Protein: 10 grams |
| Carbohydrates: 8 grams |
| Fat: 3 grams |
| Fiber: 2 grams |

Try to stick with low-fat cheese here, as regular Cheddar adds 65 calories and 8 grams of fat more per serving.

℘

# Easy Corn Chowder

1 (14-ounce) can vegetable or
   chicken broth
2 (10-ounce) bags frozen corn
   (combine white and yellow,
   if desired)
1 small potato, peeled and
   cubed

1 onion, chopped
½ teaspoon salt
½ teaspoon pepper
3½ cups low-fat milk, divided
2 tablespoons cornstarch

1. In a large saucepan or Dutch oven, combine broth, corn, potato, onion, salt, and pepper. Heat to boiling. Reduce heat and simmer 15 to 20 minutes or until potato is softened. Stir in 3 cups milk.
2. In a small bowl, combine remaining ½ cup milk with cornstarch. Add to soup over low heat until soup thickens.

| **Serves 6** |
| 1 bread, 1 vegetable, ½ dairy |
| --- |
| Calories per serving: 195 |
| Protein: 9 grams |
| Carbohydrates: 36 grams |
| Fat: 3 grams |
| Fiber: 3 grams |

You can cut down to skim milk and cut an additional 13 calories and 2 grams of fat per serving.

℘

# Orange Chicken

**Serves 4**
**1 meat, ½ fruit, 1 fat**

Calories per serving: 234

Protein: 27 grams

Carbohydrates: 18 grams

Fat: 6 grams

Fiber: 0

Watch the size of the chicken breasts. Some are actually double the size of a 3-ounce portion.

∾

*1 tablespoon margarine*
*2 garlic cloves, minced*
*4 boneless, skinless chicken*
*  breasts*
*½ teaspoon dried rosemary*

*salt and pepper to taste*
*½ cup orange juice*
*¼ cup orange marmalade*
*1 teaspoon cornstarch*

1. In large skillet, melt margarine over medium heat. Sauté garlic. Add chicken breasts, rosemary, and salt and pepper. Cook until chicken breasts begin to brown, about 3 to 4 minutes on each side. Remove chicken from skillet.
2. In a small bowl, combine orange juice, marmalade, cornstarch, and 3 tablespoons of water. Pour mixture into skillet. Heat 2 to 3 minutes, while stirring, until orange mixture begins to thicken. Add chicken back to skillet. Cover and simmer for 10 to 15 minutes.

# Chicken Dijon

**Serves 4**
**1 meat**

Calories per serving: 106

Protein: 20 grams

Carbohydrates: 2 grams

Fat: 2 grams

Fiber: 0

This simple chicken dish goes with any pasta, rice, or potato, and vegetable side dish of your choice.

∾

*4 boneless, skinless chicken*
*  breasts*
*2 teaspoons lemon juice*
*2 garlic cloves, minced*

*2 tablespoons Dijon mustard*
*½ teaspoon salt*
*½ teaspoon black pepper*

1. Preheat oven to 375 degrees.
2. Place chicken breasts in a glass baking dish. In a small bowl, combine lemon juice, garlic, mustard, salt, and pepper. Mix together. Spread mustard mixture over tops of chicken breasts. Bake 20 to 30 minutes or until chicken is done and no longer pink in the center.

# Chicken Vegetable Stir-Fry

*4 skinless, boneless chicken
   breasts*
*1 teaspoon salt*
*½ teaspoon pepper*
*1 teaspoon paprika*
*2 tablespoons flour*
*2 tablespoons oil, divided*
*½ cup chopped green onions*

*1 garlic clove, minced*
*1 cup fresh broccoli florets*
*1 red bell pepper, cut into
   strips*
*1 green bell pepper, cut into
   strips*
*½ cup chicken or vegetable
   broth*

| Serves 6 |
| --- |
| **1 meat, 1 vegetable, ½ fat** |
| Calories per serving: 136 |
| Protein: 14 grams |
| Carbohydrates: 6 grams |
| Fat: 6 grams |
| Fiber: 2 grams |

Top with ½ cup chow mein noodles and add 20 calories and 1½ grams of fat per serving.

1. Cut chicken into ½-inch strips. In a shallow dish or pie pan, combine salt, pepper, paprika, and flour. Add chicken strips to flour mixture and coat well.
2. In a large skillet, heat 1 tablespoon of the oil. Add chicken. Cook until golden brown. Remove chicken to a large plate.
3. Heat remaining tablespoon of oil. Add onion, garlic, broccoli, and peppers. Cook until vegetables are slightly tender. Return chicken to pan and add broth. Cook until thoroughly heated and about half of the broth evaporates.

# Lemon Fish Fillets with Capers

| Serves 4 |
| --- |
| 1½ meat, ½ bread, 1 fat |

| |
| --- |
| Calories per serving: 206 |
| Protein: 19 grams |
| Carbohydrates: 6 grams |
| Fat: 11 grams |
| Fiber: .5 gram |

Cook fish in 2 tablespoons of broth or use vegetable oil cooking spray instead of oil to save 60 calories and 7 grams of fat per serving.

ℭ

¼ cup flour
½ teaspoon salt
½ teaspoon pepper
1 pound fish fillets (flounder, whitefish, fillet of sole, tilapia)

2 tablespoons oil
1 teaspoon margarine
1 tablespoon capers
1 tablespoon lemon juice or 1 fresh lemon

1. In a shallow dish or pie pan, combine flour, salt, and pepper. Add fish fillets to flour mixture and coat well.
2. In a large skillet, heat oil. Cook fish until lightly browned, about 3 to 5 minutes on each side. Remove fish to serving platter.
3. Remove skillet from heat. Add margarine, capers, and lemon juice to warm skillet. Heat until margarine is just melted. Pour sauce over fish fillets to serve.

# Salmon Fettuccini

*1 pound fettuccini noodles
(can also use other pasta,
like bow ties)*
*2 tablespoons margarine*
*2 green onions, finely chopped*
*1 pound skinless salmon fillet,
cut into chunks*

*2 tablespoons lemon juice*
*salt and pepper to taste*
*1 cup frozen baby peas*
*1 teaspoon dill weed*
*2 tablespoons Parmesan cheese*

| **Serves 6** |
| :---: |
| **1 meat, 1½ bread, 1 fat** |

| |
| --- |
| Calories per serving: 280 |
| Protein: 21 grams |
| Carbohydrates: 26 grams |
| Fat: 10 grams |
| Fiber: 3 grams |

Cut the margarine in half and save 20 calories and 2 grams of fat per serving.

∾

1. Prepare pasta according to package directions. Drain.
2. In large skillet, melt margarine over medium heat. Add onions, salmon chunks, lemon juice, and salt and pepper. Cook about 3 to 5 minutes until salmon is cooked throughout and no longer opaque. Add ¼ cup water and the peas. Heat until water evaporates and peas are cooked. Toss with drained fettuccini. Sprinkle with dill and Parmesan cheese to serve.

# Lentil Spaghetti

8 ounces spaghetti noodles
1 tablespoon oil
½ onion, chopped
2 garlic cloves, minced
1 cup dry lentils
½ teaspoon thyme
½ teaspoon salt
½ teaspoon red pepper flakes
1 tomato, diced
2 ounces feta cheese
2 teaspoons parsley

1. Prepare spaghetti according to package directions. Drain.
2. In a Dutch oven, heat oil. Add onion and garlic. Cook over medium heat for about 3 minutes. Add the lentils and 1½ cups of water. Bring to a boil. Add thyme, salt, red pepper flakes, and tomatoes. Bring to boil again. Reduce heat. Simmer, uncovered, for 30 minutes until lentils are softened.
3. To serve, place spaghetti onto serving platter. Top with lentils. Sprinkle with feta cheese and parsley.

# Pasta Primavera

8 ounces linguini noodles
2 tablespoons oil
2 garlic cloves, minced
1 red bell pepper, cut into strips
1 yellow bell pepper, cut into strips
2 small zucchini, thinly sliced
4 ounces fresh snow peas, trimmed
1 pint cherry tomatoes, cut in half
1 tablespoon chopped fresh basil

1. Prepare linguini noodles according to package directions. Drain.
2. In a large skillet, heat oil. Add garlic, peppers, zucchini, and snow peas. Stir-fry vegetables until tender. Add drained pasta, cherry tomatoes, and basil. Toss.

# Sesame Noodles with Peppers & Pine Nuts

8 ounces spaghetti noodles
1 teaspoon vegetable oil
½ red bell pepper, thinly sliced
¼ cup green onions, thinly
    sliced
1 (14-ounce) can bean sprouts,
    drained
2 tablespoons fresh basil,
    chopped
1 tablespoons fresh cilantro,
    chopped
2 tablespoons pine nuts

## Dressing:

¼ cup lime juice
3 tablespoons soy sauce
1 tablespoon brown sugar
1 tablespoon water
1 tablespoon sesame oil
1 teaspoon ground ginger
2 garlic cloves, minced
dash red pepper flakes

| Serves 6 |
| --- |
| 2 bread, ½ vegetable, 1 fat |

| | |
| --- | --- |
| Calories per serving: 219 | |
| Protein: 7 grams | |
| Carbohydrates: 37 grams | |
| Fat: 4 grams | |
| Fiber: 3 grams | |

This pasta dish will jazz up your baked chicken breast or fish fillet.

∾

1. Prepare spaghetti noodles according to package directions. Drain.
2. In a large skillet, heat the vegetable oil. Add red bell pepper and onion. Sauté until slightly tender. Add drained bean sprouts and spaghetti noodles. Remove from heat. Toss with basil, cilantro, and pine nuts.
3. Combine dressing ingredients. Mix well. Pour spaghetti mixture into a large bowl. Toss with dressing. Serve slightly warm or cold.

# Chicken Vegetable Couscous

**Serves 6**
2 breads, 1 vegetable,
1 meat

Calories per serving: 255

Protein: 15 grams

Carbohydrates: 43 grams

Fat: 3 grams

Fiber: 3 grams

The small amount of feta cheese really adds to the taste of this dish. It only adds 18 calories and 1 gram of fat per serving.

ᘐ

*2 boneless, skinless chicken breasts*
*1 (10-ounce) package couscous*
*1 (14-ounce) can chicken or vegetable broth*
*3 large tomatoes, finely chopped*

*2 garlic cloves, minced*
*2 tablespoons fresh basil, finely chopped*
*2 tablespoons balsamic vinegar*
*salt and pepper to taste*
*¼ cup feta cheese, crumbled*

1. Bake, boil, or broil chicken breasts. Cool slightly. Slice into thin strips.
2. Prepare couscous according to package directions, using chicken broth in place of water. (Do not add margarine or oil as directed.)
3. When couscous is done, pour it out into a large bowl. Toss with chopped tomatoes, garlic, basil, vinegar, and salt and pepper. Add chicken strips and crumbled feta cheese on top to serve.

# Pineapple Cole Slaw

**Serves 6**
1 vegetable, ½ fat

Calories per serving: 65

Protein: 1 gram

Carbohydrates: 12 grams

Fat: 2 grams

Fiber: 2 grams

Be creative—add other vegetables to your liking too . . . red and yellow bell peppers, celery, whatever you like.

ᘐ

*4 cups cabbage, finely shredded*
*½ cup carrots, finely shredded*
*¼ cup green bell pepper, finely chopped*
*1 (12-ounce) can unsweetened crushed pineapple, drained*

*2 tablespoons low-fat mayonnaise*
*1 tablespoon rice vinegar*
*1 tablespoon brown sugar*
*1 teaspoon spicy mustard*
*salt and pepper to taste*

In a large bowl, combine cabbage, carrots, peppers, and pineapple. Mix well. In a small bowl, combine remaining ingredients. Toss dressing with vegetables. Chill until ready to serve.

# Asparagus Deluxe

*1 pound fresh asparagus spears*
*1 tablespoon olive oil*

*2 tablespoons pine nuts*
*1½ teaspoons Parmesan cheese*

1. Preheat oven to 350 degrees.
2. Cut asparagus spears into 1-inch pieces and place into a baking dish. Drizzle oil over asparagus. Toss with pine nuts and Parmesan cheese. Cook for 15 minutes or until asparagus is tender.

**Serves 6**
**1 vegetable, ½ fat**

Calories per serving: 59

Protein: 3 grams

Carbohydrates: 4 grams

Fat: 4 grams

Fiber: 2 grams

To reduce calories by 16 and fat by 1.5 grams per serving, eliminate the pine nuts.

∽

# Tossed Salad with Tomato Basil Salad Dressing

*1 head lettuce, finely torn*
*¼ cup red onion, finely chopped*

**Dressing:**

*6 sun-dried tomatoes*
*1 large tomato, finely chopped*

*2 garlic cloves, minced*
*¼ cup fresh basil, finely chopped*
*2 tablespoons balsamic vinegar*
*salt and pepper to taste*

1. Prepare salad. Place in large bowl.
2. In a small bowl, combine sun-dried tomatoes with ½ cup boiling water. Let sit aside for 3 to 5 minutes. Drain.
3. In electric blender, combine remaining ingredients and ½ cup water. Mix well. Add sun-dried tomatoes. Purée until dressing is smooth.
4. Toss salad with dressing to serve.

**Serves 6**
**1 vegetable**

Calories per serving: 29

Protein: 2 grams

Carbohydrates: 6 grams

Fat: 0

Fiber: 2 grams

Toss entire salad with 1 cup seasoned croutons for only 31 additional calories and 1 gram of fat per serving.

∽

# Cinnamon Apple Chips

*2 apples, sliced very thin*
*1 tablespoon sugar*

*1 teaspoon cinnamon*

1. Preheat oven to 200 degrees.
2. Cover a cookie sheet with parchment paper. Lay out apple slices in a single layer over the parchment paper.
3. In a small bowl, combine the sugar and cinnamon. Sprinkle over apples.
4. Bake for 1½ hours until the apple slices dry out. Remove from pan.

**Serves 4**
**½ fruit**

Calories per serving: 54

Protein: 0

Carbohydrates: 15 grams

Fat: 0

Fiber: 3 grams

Make a bunch. These go fast. Just watch how many you eat.

# Yogurt Parfait

*1 (8-ounce) carton low-fat*
  *vanilla yogurt*
*¼ cup fresh blueberries*

*¼ cup fresh raspberries*
*1 small banana, thinly sliced*
*¼ cup low-fat granola*

In two parfait or tall glasses, layer yogurt and fruit as desired. Top off with granola. Serve immediately.

**Serves 2**
**1 fruit, ½ dairy, 1 fat**

Calories per serving: 224

Protein: 7 grams

Carbohydrates: 47 grams

Fat: 2 grams

Fiber: 3 grams

Eliminate the granola to cut 40 calories and 1 gram of fat per serving.

# Watermelon Ice

*4 cups frozen watermelon
chunks, seeds removed*

*2 tablespoons sugar
1 teaspoon lemon juice*

Place all the ingredients in a blender. Purée until smooth. Serve immediately.

**Serves 4**
**1 fruit, ½ fat**

Calories per serving: 74

Protein: 1 gram

Carbohydrates: 17 grams

Fat: 0

Fiber: 1 gram

Stick to a serving size of this refreshing ice treat. It's so good, you may be tempted to eat more.

# Frozen Yogurt Sandwich

*2 graham cracker rectangles,
broken into squares*

*¼ cup low-fat frozen yogurt,
any flavor, slightly softened*

Lay graham cracker squares onto a flat surface. Top 2 squares with frozen yogurt. Place remaining squares on top to make a sandwich. Serve immediately or wrap in plastic wrap and freeze until ready to eat.

**Serves 2**
**1 bread, ½ fat**

Calories per serving: 85

Protein: 2 grams

Carbohydrates: 15 grams

Fat: 2 grams

Fiber: 0

Experiment with different flavors of frozen yogurt or sherbet for low-fat dessert treats.

# Zesty Fruit Juice

| | |
|---|---|
| **Serves 4**<br>**1 fruit** | |
| Calories per serving: 77 | |
| Protein: 1 gram | |
| Carbohydrates: 19 grams | |
| Fat: 0 | |
| Fiber: 0 | |

For an occasional treat, add ½ cup low-fat frozen yogurt to the zesty fruit juice. By doing so, you will only increase calories by 25 per serving.

∾

2 cups sparkling water

2 cups grape, cranberry, orange, or other juice of choice

In a pitcher, combine sparkling water with juice. Mix well to serve.

# Cinnamon Baked Apples

| | |
|---|---|
| **Serves 4**<br>**1½ fruit** | |
| Calories: 128 | |
| Protein: 1 gram | |
| Carbohydrates: 34 grams | |
| Fat: 0 | |
| Fiber: 3.5 grams | |

Place apples in the oven just before you sit down to dinner. They will be ready as a treat following the meal.

∾

4 tart yellow apples, like Granny Smith
2 tablespoons honey
1 tablespoon lemon juice

2 teaspoons cinnamon
½ teaspoon nutmeg
1 cup apple juice

1. Preheat oven to 375 degrees. Wash apples. Remove center core without cutting all the way through the apple. Place apples in a small baking dish.
2. In small bowl, combine honey, lemon juice, cinnamon, and nutmeg. Divide the mixture and place into the center of each apple. Pour apple juice over and around the apples.
3. Bake 35 to 45 minutes or until apples are soft. Be sure to baste apples occasionally, every 10 to 15 minutes.

# Toss It up Trail Mix

2 cups toasted oat cereal
1 cup pretzel sticks
1 cup small oyster crackers
$\frac{1}{2}$ cup dry-roasted peanuts
$\frac{1}{2}$ cup sunflower seeds, shelled

$\frac{1}{2}$ cup raisins
$\frac{1}{2}$ cup semisweet chocolate
  chips

In a large bowl, combine all ingredients. Mix or shake well. Store in air-tight container.

**Yields 24 $\frac{1}{4}$-cup servings**

**1$\frac{1}{2}$ bread, $\frac{1}{2}$ fat**

| | |
|---|---|
| Calories: 175 | |
| Protein: 4 grams | |
| Carbohydrates: 29 grams | |
| Fat: 5 grams | |
| Fiber: 2 grams | |

A combination of many snack foods can make a favorite trail mix. Play around with dry cereals, dried fruits, crackers, and nuts.

# Chocolate Chip Meringue Bites

2 large egg whites
$\frac{1}{2}$ teaspoon cream of tartar
$\frac{3}{4}$ cup sugar

$\frac{3}{4}$ cup mini semisweet or milk
  chocolate chips

1. Preheat oven to 200 degrees. Line a cookie sheet with parchment paper.
2. In medium mixing bowl, beat egg whites and cream of tartar with electric mixer until foamy. Slowly add sugar. Continue beating at high speed until stiff peaks form.
3. Use a wooden spoon or rubber spatula to fold the chocolate chips into the meringue.
4. Drop meringue by tablespoonfuls onto parchment paper.
5. Bake 1$\frac{1}{2}$ hours. Remove from oven. Cool before removing from parchment paper. Store in airtight container.

**Yields 3 dozen**
**1 extra (sugar)**

| | |
|---|---|
| Calories: 34 | |
| Protein: 0 | |
| Carbohydrates: 6 grams | |
| Fat: 1 gram | |
| Fiber: 0 | |

These bites are sure to satisfy any sweet tooth.

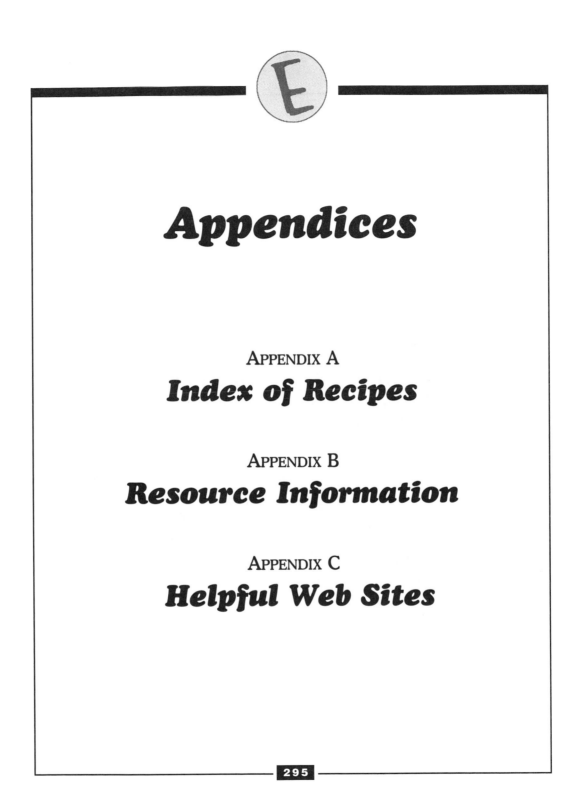

# *Appendices*

APPENDIX A
## *Index of Recipes*

APPENDIX B
## *Resource Information*

APPENDIX C
## *Helpful Web Sites*

# APPENDIX A
# *Index of Recipes*

# APPENDIX B
# *Resource Information*

## Contact Information for Resources

American Dietetic Association
216 West Jackson Boulevard
Chicago, IL 60606
Phone: 800-366-1655
Web site: *www.eatright.org*

International Food Information
Council
1100 Connecticut Avenue NW,
Suite 430
Washington, D.C. 20036
Phone: 202-296-6540
Web site: *www.ific.org*

Food and Nutrition Service
USDA
3101 Park Center Drive
Alexandria, VA 22302
Web site: *www.fns.usda.gov/fns*

Food and Drug Administration
200 C Street SW
Washington, D.C. 20204
Web site: *www.fda.gov*

Food Safety and Inspection
Service
USDA
1400 Independence Avenue, SW
Room 2942S
Washington, D.C. 20250
Web site: *www.fsis.usda.gov*

Food Safety Information
Web site: *www.foodsafety.gov*

National Eating Disorders
Association
603 Stewart Street, Suite 803
Seattle, WA 98101
Phone: 206-382-3587
Web site:
*www.nationaleatingdisorders.org*

National Association of Anorexia
Nervosa and Associated Disorders
P.O. Box 7
Highland Park, IL 60035
Phone: 847-831-3438
Web site: *www.anad.org*

Anorexia Nervosa and Related
Eating Disorders (ANRED)
P.O. Box 5102
Eugene, OR 97405
Phone: 541-344-1144
Web site: *www.anred.com*

President's Council on Physical
Fitness and Sports
Department W
200 Independence Avenue, SW
Room 738-H
Washington, D.C. 20201-0004
Phone: 202-690-9000
Web site: *www.fitness.gov*

American College of Sports
Medicine
P.O. Box 1440
Indianapolis, IN 46206-1440
Phone: 317-637-9200
Web site: *www.acsm.org*

Weight-control Information
Network
1 WIN Way
Bethesda, MD 20892-3665
Phone: 202-828-1025 or
877-WIN-4627
Web site: *www.niddk.nih.gov/
health/nutrit/win.htm*

National Health Information
Center
U.S. Department of Health and
Human Services
P.O. Box 1133
Washington, D.C. 20013-1133
Web site: *www.healthfinder.gov*

National Heart, Lung, and Blood
Institute Information Center
P.O. Box 30101
Bethesda, MD 20824-0105
Web site: *www.nhlbi.nih.gov*

# Appendix C
# *Helpful Web Sites*

- *www.cyberdiet.com*: Offers helpful information for weight-loss success, including eating right, exercising smart, and feeling good.

- *www.phys.com:* Offers tips and articles on staying fit, eating well, and being happy.

- *www.aerobics.com:* Official site of the Aerobics and Fitness Association of America that offers information for fitness professionals and exercise enthusiasts alike.

- *www.oxygen.com/topic/health:* Interactive site that brings diet and nutrition, health and fitness information to users.

- *www.niddk.nih.gov:* From the National Institute of Diabetes and Digestive and Kidney Disorders, offering health, weight-loss and control information, research, and educational materials.

- *www.caloriecontrol.org:* Provides information on reducing overall fat and caloric intake and achieving and maintaining a healthy weight.

- *www.thedietchannel.com:* Offers helpful tips on successful weight loss, analyzing diets, nutrition information, and more.

- *www.weightfocus.com:* Shares a collection of articles, diet and health information, weight-loss strategies, and more to help users achieve success in weight reduction and exercise.

# Index

# THE EVERYTHING TOTAL FITNESS BOOK

## By Ellen Karpay

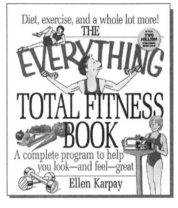

The Everything® Total Fitness Book features complete information and instructions on the best exercises for aerobic and muscular fitness, from outdoor sports to the latest machines at the gym. The step-by-step illustrations of exercise, weight training, and stretching techniques will help ensure that your workouts are safe and effective. With dozens of helpful hints, tips, and excuse-busters, you'll quickly develop a routine that works for you. You'll learn to build time for rigorous and effective exercise into even the busiest schedule.

Trade paperback, $12.95
1-58062-318-2, 304 pages

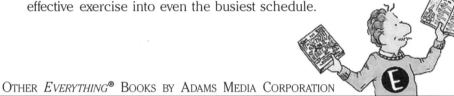

OTHER *EVERYTHING*® BOOKS BY ADAMS MEDIA CORPORATION

Everything® **After College Book**
$12.95, 1-55850-847-3

Everything® **American History Book**
$12.95, 1-58062-531-2

Everything® **Angels Book**
$12.95, 1-58062-398-0

Everything® **Anti-Aging Book**
$12.95, 1-58062-565-7

Everything® **Astrology Book**
$14.95, 1-58062-062-0

Everything® **Astronomy Book**
$14.95, 1-58062-723-4

Everything® **Baby Names Book**
$12.95, 1-55850-655-1

Everything® **Baby Shower Book**
$12.95, 1-58062-305-0

Everything® **Baby's First Food Book**
$12.95, 1-58062-512-6

Everything® **Baby's First Year Book**
$12.95, 1-58062-581-9

Everything® **Barbecue Cookbook**
$14.95, 1-58062-316-6

Everything® **Bartender's Book**
$9.95, 1-55850-536-9

Everything® **Bedtime Story Book**
$12.95, 1-58062-147-3

Everything® **Bible Stories Book**
$14.95, 1-58062-547-9

Everything® **Bicycle Book**
$12.00, 1-55850-706-X

Everything® **Breastfeeding Book**
$12.95, 1-58062-582-7

Everything® **Budgeting Book**
$14.95, 1-58062-786-2

Everything® **Build Your Own Home Page Book**
$12.95, 1-58062-339-5

Everything® **Business Planning Book**
$12.95, 1-58062-491-X

Everything® **Candlemaking Book**
$12.95, 1-58062-623-8

Everything® **Car Care Book**
$14.95, 1-58062-732-3

Everything® **Casino Gambling Book**
$12.95, 1-55850-762-0

Everything® **Cat Book**
$12.95, 1-55850-710-8

Everything® **Chocolate Cookbook**
$12.95, 1-58062-405-7

Everything® **Christmas Book**
$15.00, 1-55850-697-7

Everything® **Civil War Book**
$12.95, 1-58062-366-2

Everything® **Classical Mythology Book**
$12.95, 1-58062-653-X

Everything® **Coaching & Mentoring Book**
$14.95, 1-58062-730-7

Everything® **Collectibles Book**
$12.95, 1-58062-645-9

Everything® **College Survival Book**
$14.95, 1-55850-720-5

Everything® **Computer Book**
$12.95, 1-58062-401-4

Everything® **Cookbook**
$14.95, 1-58062-400-6

Everything® **Cover Letter Book**
$14.95, 1-58062-312-3

Everything® **Creative Writing Book**
$14.95, 1-58062-647-5

Everything® **Crossword and Puzzle Book**
$14.95, 1-55850-764-7

Everything® **Dating Book**
$12.95, 1-58062-185-6

Everything® **Pregnancy Organizer**
$15.00, 1-58062-336-0

Everything® **Project Management Book**
$12.95, 1-58062-583-5

Everything® **Puppy Book**
$12.95, 1-58062-576-2

Everything® **Quick Meals Cookbook**
$14.95, 1-58062-488-X

Everything® **Resume Book**
$12.95, 1-58062-311-5

Everything® **Romance Book**
$12.95, 1-58062-566-5

Everything® **Running Book**
$12.95, 1-58062-618-1

Everything® **Sailing Book, 2nd Ed.**
$12.95, 1-58062-671-8

Everything® **Saints Book**
$12.95, 1-58062-534-7

Everything® **Scrapbooking Book**
$14.95, 1-58062-729-3

Everything® **Selling Book**
$12.95, 1-58062-319-0

Everything® **Shakespeare Book**
$14.95, 1-58062-591-6

Everything® **Slow Cooker Cookbook**
$14.95, 1-58062-667-X

Everything® **Soup Cookbook**
$14.95, 1-58062-556-8

Everything® **Spells and Charms Book**
$12.95, 1-58062-532-0

Everything® **Start Your Own Business Book**
$14.95, 1-58062-650-5

Everything® **Stress Management Book**
$14.95, 1-58062-578-9

Everything® **Study Book**
$12.95, 1-55850-615-2

Everything® **T'ai Chi and QiGong Book**
$12.95, 1-58062-646-7

Everything® **Tall Tales, Legends, and Other Outrageous Lies Book**
$12.95, 1-58062-514-2

Everything® **Tarot Book**
$12.95, 1-58062-191-0

Everything® **Thai Cookbook**
$14.95, 1-58062-733-1

Everything® **Time Management Book**
$12.95, 1-58062-492-8

Everything® **Toasts Book**
$12.95, 1-58062-189-9

Everything® **Toddler Book**
$14.95, 1-58062-592-4

Everything® **Total Fitness Book**
$12.95, 1-58062-318-2

Everything® **Trivia Book**
$12.95, 1-58062-143-0

Everything® **Tropical Fish Book**
$12.95, 1-58062-343-3

Everything® **Vegetarian Cookbook**
$12.95, 1-58062-640-8

Everything® **Vitamins, Minerals, and Nutritional Supplements Book**
$12.95, 1-58062-496-0

Everything® **Weather Book**
$14.95, 1-58062-668-8

Everything® **Wedding Book, 2nd Ed.**
$14.95, 1-58062-190-2

Everything® **Wedding Checklist**
$7.95, 1-58062-456-1

Everything® **Wedding Etiquette Book**
$7.95, 1-58062-454-5

Everything® **Wedding Organizer**
$15.00, 1-55850-828-7

Everything® **Wedding Shower Book**
$7.95, 1-58062-188-0

Everything® **Wedding Vows Book**
$7.95, 1-58062-455-3

Everything® **Weddings on a Budget Book**
$9.95, 1-58062-782-X

Everything® **Weight Training Book**
$14.95, 1-58062-593-2

Everything® **Wicca and Witchcraft Book**
$14.95, 1-58062-725-0

Everything® **Wine Book**
$12.95, 1-55850-808-2

Everything® **World War II Book**
$14.95, 1-58062-572-X

Everything® **World's Religions Book**
$14.95, 1-58062-648-3

Everything® **Yoga Book**
$14.95, 1-58062-594-0

*Prices subject to change without notice.

# EVERYTHING® **KIDS'** SERIES!

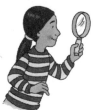

Everything® **Kids' Baseball Book, 2nd Ed.**
$6.95, 1-58062-688-2

Everything® **Kids' Cookbook**
$6.95, 1-58062-658-0

Everything® **Kids' Joke Book**
$6.95, 1-58062-686-6

Everything® **Kids' Mazes Book**
$6.95, 1-58062-558-4

Everything® **Kids' Money Book**
$6.95, 1-58062-685-8

Everything® **Kids' Monsters Book**
$6.95, 1-58062-657-2

Everything® **Kids' Nature Book**
$6.95, 1-58062-684-X

Everything® **Kids' Puzzle Book**
$6.95, 1-58062-687-4

Everything® **Kids' Science Experiments Book**
$6.95, 1-58062-557-6

Everything® **Kids' Soccer Book**
$6.95, 1-58062-642-4

Everything® **Kids' Travel Activity Book**
$6.95, 1-58062-641-6

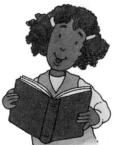

## Available wherever books are sold!
## To order, call 800-872-5627, or visit us at everything.com

Everything® is a registered trademark of Adams Media Corporation.